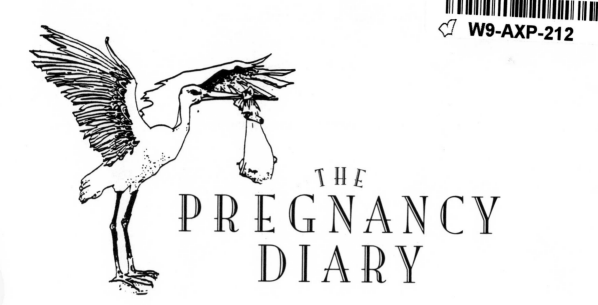

THE PREGNANCY DIARY

TRACIE HOTCHNER

Illustrated by Christine Perry

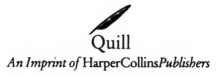

Quill
An Imprint of HarperCollinsPublishers

Other Books for Expectant Parents

by Tracie Hotchner

PREGNANCY & CHILDBIRTH
PREGNANCY PURE & SIMPLE

Special thanks to Alison Levant

HarperCollins books may be purchased for educational, business, or sales promotional use. For information please write: Special Markets Department, HarperCollins Publishers Inc., 10 East 53rd Street, New York, NY 10022.

First Avon paperback edition published 1992.

Reprinted in Quill 2002.

Library of Congress Cataloging- in -Publication Data

Hotchner, Tracie.
The pregnancy diary / Tracie Hotchner; illustrated by Christine Perry.
  p. cm.
  1. Pregnancy—popular works. I. Title.
RG525.H583   1992   92-22580
618.2'4—dc20   CIP

ISBN 0-380-76543-8

04 05 06 QW 20 19 18 17

My due date is _____

My obstetrician's name is _____

My midwife or nurse-midwife's name is _____

My Lamaze teacher's name is _____

I'm expecting to give birth at _____

I know I'm going to have a _____

The baby's pediatrician will be _____

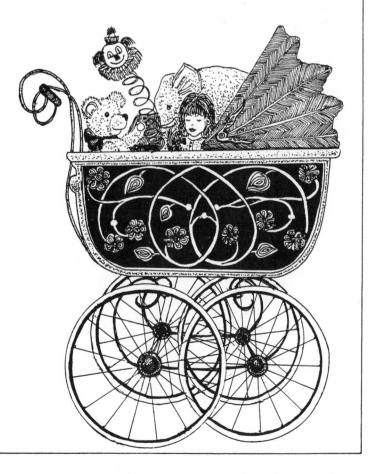

Welcome to Your Pregnancy Diary!

Make yourself at home . . . . because this diary is going to be an emotional home for you during the adventure of your pregnancy. This isn't a traditional book that you sit and read: it needs *you* to make it come alive. This diary needs you to breathe life into it and nourish it, much like the baby inside you. Without your special touch, this book is an empty shell. This diary is an invitation to get to know yourself better. It's a chance to chronicle your personal experience of pregnancy along with your baby's earliest history. In all the excitement about the developments inside your belly, it's easy to overlook what's going on in your heart and mind. This diary is a place to explore and celebrate your emotional and imaginative sides as a mother-to-be.

You may have picked up this book because you recognized my name as the author of *Pregnancy & Childbirth* and *Childbirth & Marriage.* Those books gave encyclopedic attention to facts, to theories, to everything the pregnant woman and couple needs to know. But sometimes you need a break from the avalanche of information that overtakes you when you're expecting. Pregnancy is a time when it may seem as though everyone is telling you what you should or shouldn't eat or drink, where you can't go, what you must do. I don't want this to be one more finger wagging at you, telling you what is bad for your baby, what to avoid, what to worry about, and so on. This diary is a place to get away from all that, to explore your feelings, to dream your dreams, to indulge yourself. Enjoy this diary as your special place to escape from the practical concerns of being pregnant and allow yourself to get caught up in your fantasies and feelings.

This book was born from the desire to help you connect to that personal aspect of being pregnant, get in touch with the emotional highs and lows, keep track of milestones, and hold on to these memories. The diary is aimed at your heart and mind, at the vulnerability and openness that are part of being pregnant. You can transform all these feelings into a memento of the precious months while you await your child. You may feel overwhelmed by colliding emotions, by changes you are undergoing. This diary is where you can bring all that excitement and turn it into something to treasure years from now (when your toddler is throwing mashed beets at the wall, or your preteenager is being a hormonal terrorist!). I want to encourage you to be contemplative, imaginative, romantic, and playful about your unborn child. Years from now, this book will be a keepsake—one you may even want to share with your child so he or she can discover the intense, intimate, wonderful moments you had during the first nine months.

What About Starting the Diary Late?

If you are three or four months along in your pregnancy before you start keeping this diary, don't ignore those early months that may have already gone by. When you have time, you might want to go back and fill in the early weeks of the diary, remembering details as well as you can. You'll enjoy putting into perspective what you were feeling and thinking in those early weeks and months. If you're willing to take the time to backtrack and fill in the gaps, you'll have a more complete diary of your pregnancy. You'll also get the unusual chance to relive the earliest time in your baby's growth.

How the Diary Is Organized

The diary is divided into one-week intervals, with repeating pages described in detail on the following pages. At close to monthly intervals, or that point in your pregnancy when you'll probably be seeing your obstetrician, you'll find a page to record your doctor visit.

After your baby is born, you'll find special pages designed to let you finish up your diary with a record of your passage into parenthood. "Life After Birth—The First Month" and the two sections that follow are a private place for you to continue paying attention to yourself and to what having a baby has meant to you.

There are also specialized pages for particular points in your pregnancy, such as "My Baby Shower," "My Childbirth Class," and "Secrets of My Bag for the Hospital!" Finally, at the back of your diary you'll find information on your baby's astrological sign.

There may be times when you feel self-conscious or lazy about filling in the pages of the diary—but you'll kick yourself later if you don't make that little extra effort on days when you'd rather just skip it!

What You'll Find Every Week

The diary is divided by weeks, with repeating pages you'll come to know well and additional, rotating, fill-in-yourself sections.

"Your Growing Baby"

Each week (through Week 39) you'll find incredible information about the new life forming inside you on the "Your Growing Baby" page. Every week brings extraordinary growth and change, and it's thrilling to know exactly what's going on "in there" as the weeks pass! You can use the space that remains on that page to jot down things you've read that mean something special to you, or even write things you'd like to say now to your growing baby.

"My Thoughts" and Questions

Throughout the diary you'll find blank sections under the heading "My Thoughts," giving you the freedom to jot down any notes, feelings, doodles, or drawings you'd like.

There will also be a personal question. Sometimes you may just want to use the question as a springboard to get you started thinking and get in touch with yourself. You should feel free to write about anything you would like, whether or not you address the particular question.

You'll find some questions have been designed to help you start thinking about the way pregnancy has brought about changes in yourself and your partner. Recognizing feelings about your relationship as you make the important, exciting transition to parenthood is the best way to keep your marriage strong and healthy.

"My Dreams"

Dreams tend to be more vivid and memorable when you are pregnant, so every week there will be a place for you to keep a dream journal. There are many reasons that dreams are stimulated when you're expecting a baby. Your subconscious can be stirred up by hopes and fears about childbirth, motherhood, your marriage, and of course, the baby. All this excitement and stress, the adjustments and inner conflicts, can surface during sleep. Preoccupations about your abilities as a mother and about the normalcy and well-being of the baby are the stuff of which pregnancy dreams are made. (Fathers-to-be can also experience bizarre or puzzling dreams.)

Increased Awareness of Dreams

At any time of stress or upheaval in a person's life, she may be more aware of dreaming. The changes she's going through are often reflected in her dreams. This is particularly true of pregnancy, which, in addition to the mental process, also brings about powerful physical changes. The changes in your hormone levels may also be responsible for more frequent dreaming, and for dreams that seem more vivid with memorable details. You may find that you also remember more of your dreams for the simple reason that you awaken more frequently to go to the bathroom or due to other pregnancy-related discomforts. Scientific studies have shown that frequent awakening means better recall of dreams, especially if you awaken during the REM (rapid eye movement) period of sleep.

Nightmares

At some point in your pregnancy you may find that disturbing dreams outweigh the positive ones. Some nightmares may even be scary enough to awaken you. If you find that you do have dreams that are intense or frightening, *Don't worry about it!!* Seemingly out-of-control, even monstrous, dreams are considered a healthy way to express deep dreads and fears. These nighttime adventures are a normal aspect of pregnancy. Nightmares have nothing to do with what is actually going to happen. Bad dreams can be a healthy way for your mind to rid itself of its fears. Dreams with disturbing symbols or events (a funeral, snakes, an abnormal baby, giving birth to puppies) *do not foretell anything.* Don't allow yourself to get superstitious or to tell your dreams to anyone whose emotional reactions might alarm you.

Some Common Fears in Dreams
During Pregnancy

Expectant mothers (and fathers) often dream that the baby will be deformed or die, that they'll lose their partner, be a poor parent, have financial problems, or have a difficult labor and delivery.

Dreams are one way that your unconscious mind explores all the changing emotions that pregnancy stirs up. Dreams are messages sent by your inner self—you can even think of them as a secret passageway to your hidden thoughts. They are a reflection of your adjustment to pregnancy and motherhood. Your concerns, excitement, doubts, fears, and hopes emerge when you are dreaming. The dream world gives you a chance to explore your feelings about your body, your own mother, your marriage, the baby, and labor and delivery. Think of using your dreams to strengthen yourself in getting to know yourself better. Don't panic or be judgmental about fearful feelings you may have.

Of course, this isn't to say that you won't also have delightful dreams about your new life as a family, with feelings of love and warmth toward the baby you are expecting! Just keep in mind that bad dreams are nothing more than that—something you wake up from and go on to real life.

Symbols and Imagery in Dreams

Images of water or tidal waves are often found in pregnant women's dreams. Those who believe dreams are symbolic have interpreted these symbols as representing the amniotic fluid. You may also have architectural images in your dreams like tunnels, houses, boats, cars, or buildings. These symbols have been said to represent your body. Cuddly creatures or baby animals like rabbits, kittens, puppies, often appear in pregnant women's dreams. These images can be considered representational of the baby.

Remembering Your Dreams

If you awaken two or three times a night it may enable you to recall more of your dreams. However, frequent awakening is not enough to ensure that in the morning you'll remember the dreams, or the details that interest you. Recalling your dreams is something you can train yourself to do; it's a habit you can develop like any other skill. Because you need to write down the dream as soon as possible, keep this diary by your bedside. (You might prefer to scribble down your dreams on a pad of paper and transfer them later to the diary, when you might write more neatly and be more selective about what you record.)

The first thing you can do to improve your memory of dreams is to use the power of suggestion. Right before falling asleep, say to yourself, "I will remember my dreams when I wake up." When you are relaxed during sleeping, giving yourself a command like this functions as what is called a *posthypnotic suggestion* and carries a lot of weight with the subconscious.

When you wake up from the dream, remain lying still in the same position, with your eyes closed. Allow yourself to stay in a sleepy state and recall the details of the dream. In order to remember and record your dreams, it's essential that you have time to wake up gradually so you can reflect. When the dream is firmly in your mind, you can sit up slowly to write down the dream. Allow yourself to stay in a sleepy state and as relaxed as possible for the best possible recall. If you can remember only a fragment of a dream, you may find it's worthwhile to record only that portion. Recalling your dreams is a skill that will improve the more you practice it; after a few days it can become an automatic habit.

Rotating Once-a-Month Pages

"Names and Nicknames"

Once every four weeks you'll find the "Names and Nicknames" box. This is a place to keep track of funny nicknames you, your husband, or even other people close to you may be calling the baby right now. This is also a place to jot down names you are considering giving to the baby once she or he arrives.

When you are picking a name, consider that symmetry, either in the sounds or syllables, can make a first and last name sound good together. A name will often fit best with your last name if there are similar vowel or consonant sounds, or combinations of letters that repeat. For example, Grant Beltran, Travis Beltran, Vanessa Beltran, or Rebecca Beltran. As you can see, the letters don't have to be in the same order for the similar sounds to tie the names together.

Maybe you've already decided to name your baby after a family member . . . or maybe you want a traditional name like Ann or David. On the other hand, you might be eager to find a name that is unique and distinctive. If you're comfortable with an unconventional name, you might want to consider using a surname as a first name. Although surnames may at first appear to be more masculine, there are many last names that can work just as well for a girl. You can find a unique name for your baby by using your maiden name or that of one of your relatives. If you have a cumbersome family name, you can also use just part of it, so that "Brandenburg" could become "Branden." A family surname maintains a link to the past, and in the process of uncovering names, you may also learn new things about your families' histories.

Another way to find a surname to use as a first name is to think of the last names of historical figures or famous people whom you admire. For example, "Truman" could be a first name, or the *last* names of actors whose talents you admire (Gary Cooper, Bill Cosby, Robert Mitchum) might suit your baby.

Have fun with finding the baby's name—let your imagination go, and you may find your baby's name in the most unlikely place. It's fun to experiment with different names, trying them out on your spouse. Jot down the names you are considering in the special box for each monthly interval. It can be fun to look back later on the names you passed up and show them to your child years from now. ("You were almost called "Winston!")

"Getting to Know My Baby"

Once every four weeks, starting in the third month, you'll find the heading "Getting to Know My Baby." Expectant mothers have oftentimes felt their babies reacting to many things, and there is scientific evidence to suggest that your unborn baby is active, has feelings, may be sensitive to your moods, and can be aware of things going on outside your womb. If you want to keep notes now, it will give you an interesting record of your unborn baby's earliest reactions. Keeping a record of the baby's pre-birth experience may mean a lot to all of you years from now, when you or your child may want to look back at what she was like when she was "on the inside"!

"Food Cravings"

Pregnancy is rumored to bring out the desire for unusual foods at unusual times. Once a month you'll have the "pickles and ice cream" box in which you can keep notes about the strange and wonderful foods you may have been craving during that month of your pregnancy. Some women desire nothing more exotic than mashed potatoes; others crave anchovy pizzas! The "Food Cravings" box is also a good place to keep a record of those foods which, on the contrary, you can no longer stand even to see or smell, much less eat!

"Old Wives' Tales and Advice"

Why is it that people feel compelled to give a pregnant woman advice and to make comments about her condition? You'll find the "Old Wives' Tales and Advice" box at four-week intervals in the diary, where you can jot down these comments. When someone gives you some counsel you'd like to remember, or says something incredibly dumb or irritating, you may enjoy writing it down. You'll find some old wives' tales already in the diary to which you can add any superstitions and comments that you hear.

The Monthly Doctor Visit Chart

Every month (except for the second) you'll find two pages for your doctor visit, with space for you to record information you've received, and your reactions to it. Your visits to the obstetrician are not precisely monthly—you go less frequently in the first trimester and more frequently in the last trimester—but you'll find the "Doctor Visit" pages in the diary at the points during your pregnancy when appointments are normally scheduled. Each time you go for your prenatal exam you can keep a record of your thoughts and milestones as the pregnancy progresses.

You'll probably make your first prenatal visit to the doctor when you learn you're pregnant, presumably sometime in the first three months of pregnancy. After this initial doctor visit, you'll probably make monthly appointments from the twelfth week of pregnancy until the thirty-sixth week. (Of course, you'll go more frequently if you have any special problems.) Some obstetricians have a slightly different schedule for routine prenatal exams and expect their patients to make biweekly visits from the thirty-second week until the thirty-sixth. By the ninth month, an obstetrician usually expects his or her patients to come in on a weekly basis.

There will be a space for special comments or instructions from your medical care givers, as well as a place for you to make a note of any questions that you might want to ask of them when you have your appointment.

What follows is a description of what you will find on the two pages of your monthly visit to your obstetrician.

Gaining Weight

It's impossible to have a baby without gaining both weight and inches, but our society is so obsessed with weight gain that pregnant women are frequently concerned about gaining too much weight. It's good to be realistic about how and where you gain when you're expecting. From about the twelfth week of pregnancy, you'll probably notice a substantial change on the scales. If you are eating sensibly, most of the weight you are gaining (about 40 percent of it for most women) is the baby. Your increased blood volume accounts for about 22 percent of the gain, with your enhanced breasts responsible for about 8 percent, and the uterus, amniotic fluid, and placenta each accounting for 10 percent.

You'll find a place on the "Doctor Visit" page to note both your weight at that time, and how much more it is than your usual (nonpregnant) weight.

Fundal Height

You will also find a space to record your fundal height after each doctor visit. This is the distance from the top of your womb to your pubic bone, a measurement your doctor, or the nurse, will take each time that you have an appointment. The fundal height of your uterus will equal approximately the number of weeks of your pregnancy: at twenty-four weeks your fundal height will be about twenty-four centimeters.

Blood Pressure

A pregnant woman's blood pressure is measured at every visit to ensure that everything is well. If there is a rise in your blood pressure, it could be a sign of problems that your physician can then handle.

Urine

Your urine is also tested for normalcy: the presence of sugar or protein in your urine would be a sign of possible problems that the doctor will correct.

My Disappearing Waist

Every month there will be a special space for you to record the growing dimensions of your tummy. When you're pregnant, you often think about how many pounds you're gaining. You may find it more interesting to keep tabs on the changing dimensions of the middle of your body . . . that gradually "disappearing" waist! There is a space to jot down how many inches around you are at the time of each doctor visit, as well as to note how many inches you've added since the previous month.

Thigh Measurement

There is a way to check on how much superfluous body fat you are adding to your body (and will have to deal with after the baby is born). You can put a tape measure around your upper thigh and keep a record of that measurement. The circumference should actually stay the same throughout most of your pregnancy, although you should allow for more fluid retention later in the pregnancy. Be sure that you measure the same thigh each time (one may be bigger than the other to start with), and be sure that you have the tape around your leg in exactly the same position each time. You won't get an accurate measurement if you sit down one time and stand up the next. There's a space in each monthly doctor visit to record your thigh measurement, but obviously there's no need to do this; it's something you should do only if it intrigues you.

Tummy Photo

On the second page of each "Doctor Visit" entry, you'll find a framed space in which you can place a photograph of your tummy. You may find it fun to keep a record of your growing belly; the framed space is roughly the size of a Polaroid photo. If you aren't too camera-shy to take a snapshot of your stomach, it can be wonderful proof (and an astonishing reminder later on) of how your tummy ballooned as the baby grew. If you feel bold, you might want to take the picture of your belly naked; if you're modest, you may feel more comfortable wearing clothing that fits snugly over your stomach. Either way, you'll appreciate having it later on even if a monthly picture may seem foolish to you at the time. Once your pregnancy is really showing, it can be amazing to look back and see how small your stomach was just a few months before! And after your baby is born, it's incredible to see just how gigantic you were in that ninth month! You can also use this page to paste in Polaroids of ultrasound tests you might have.

Effacement and Dilation

Starting around your ninth month, or the thirty-sixth week of your pregnancy, your cervix may start to open up slowly in preparation for birth. Effacement, which is the thinning out of the cervix as it stretches, and dilation, which is the gradual opening of the cervix, are two aspects to this process. From the thirty-sixth week onward, your medical care givers may begin checking for this process; and you'll find a place to record this in your "Doctor Visit" pages.

Special Pages

You will find special sections throughout the diary, like "My Baby Shower," "My Childbirth Class," and "Secrets of My Bag for the Hospital!" along with "My Tour of the Hospital," "A Record of My Labor and Delivery," and "Baby's Day of Birth Memories." And then, because pregnancy is only the beginning of a brand-new life for you, you'll also find three special sections at the end of the diary to keep a record of the first three months of your new life as a mom and as a family. Last of all, you'll find a page with a "family tree" for a photo of your newborn babe alongside frames in which you can put photos of yourself and the baby's father when you were babies, which should be pretty cute!

Your Baby's Astrological Sign

At the end of the diary you'll find a section on the mythology of birthstones and on the signs and gems of the zodiac. You may take as fact or fantasy the information about what an astrological symbol may signify about a baby born under that sun sign, but in any case, it's fun to read about the effects that some people think the planets can have on a child's personality.

A Final Thought

The more of yourself you put into this diary, the more that you open up and let your thoughts and feelings pour out, the more precious it will be as a keepsake for you in years to come.

Your Growing Baby

Once the egg and sperm unite, the cells begin dividing, traveling along your fallopian tube until they reach your uterus, around the fourth day after fertilization. Then they multiply into what is called the blastocyst, a round, solid, growing mass of about one hundred cells. The outer layer of the blastocyst will become the placenta. The inner layer will become what is known as the embryo, once the cells have specialized into what later will be their different functions.

My Thoughts

OLD WIVES' TALES AND ADVICE

If you want a boy, stick a knife under the mattress.
If you want a girl, place a skillet under the bed.

I first realized I was pregnant when . . .

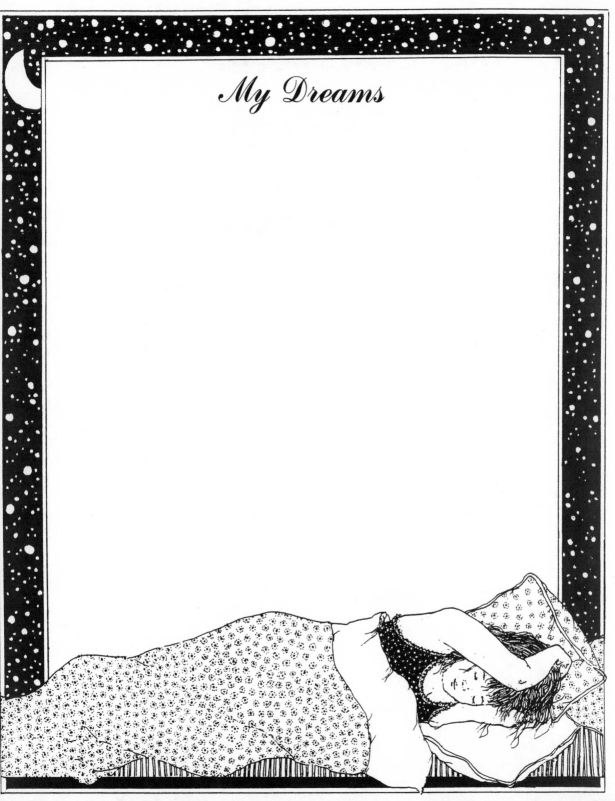

My Dreams

Your Growing Baby

In the second week, there are 150 cells that make up the embryo. The cells are divided into three layers of tissue that will develop separately. The inside layer will become the breathing and digestive organs; the middle layer is going to develop into bones, cartilage, muscles, the circulatory system, kidneys, and sex organs; the outside layer will become your baby's skin and nerves.

During this second week, the embryo floats freely in your uterus, nourished by secretions from the uterine lining.

My Thoughts

Names and Nicknames

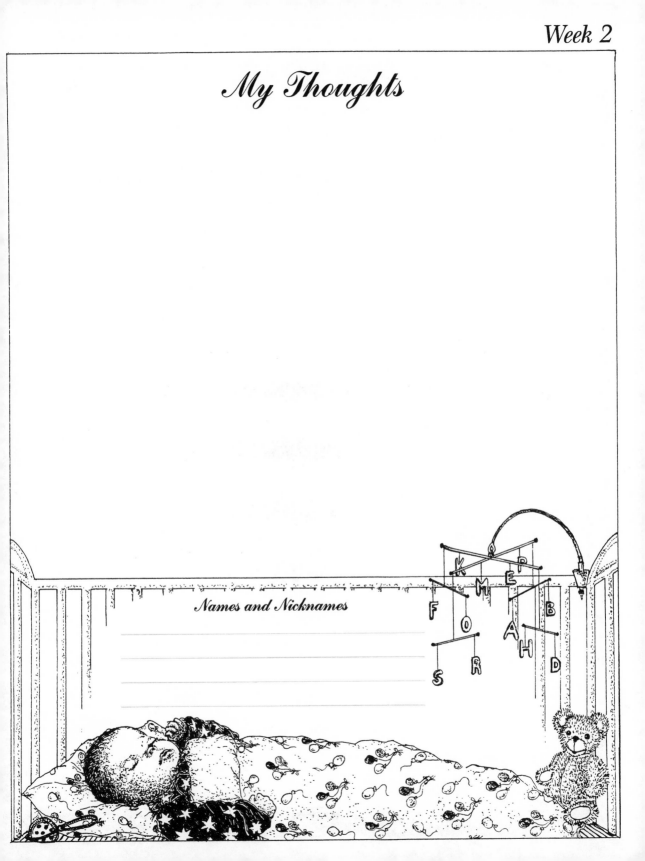

Did I choose a special way to tell my husband we were going to have a baby? Was his reaction what I expected it to be?

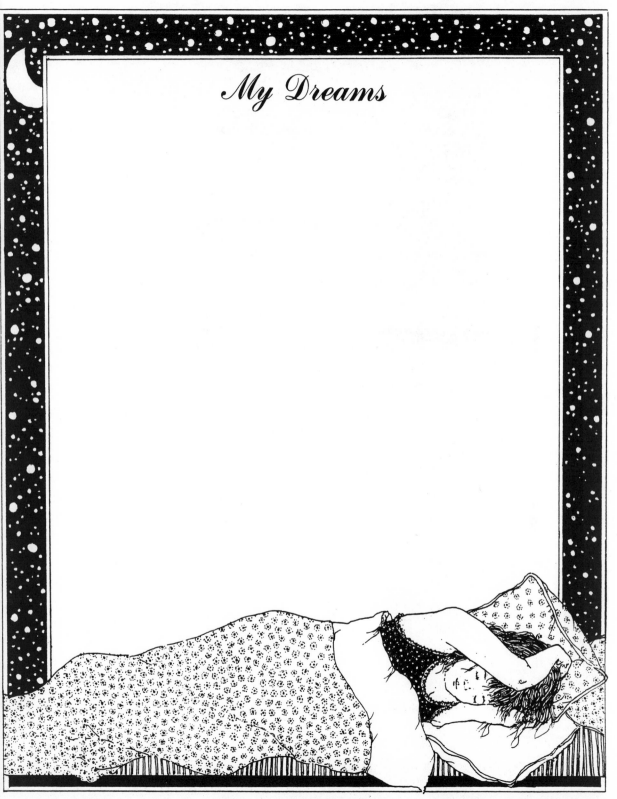

My Dreams

Your Growing Baby

By the end of the third week, the embryo begins to attach to the wall of your uterus.

The preliminary tissues are transformed into a tubular, folded structure with the beginnings of a heart, brain, and spinal cord. The outer cells surrounding the embryo spread out like roots into your uterine lining.

The deepest cells form the basis of what will become the placenta, which will nourish the baby, while other cells are developing into the amniotic sac, which will surround it.

My Thoughts

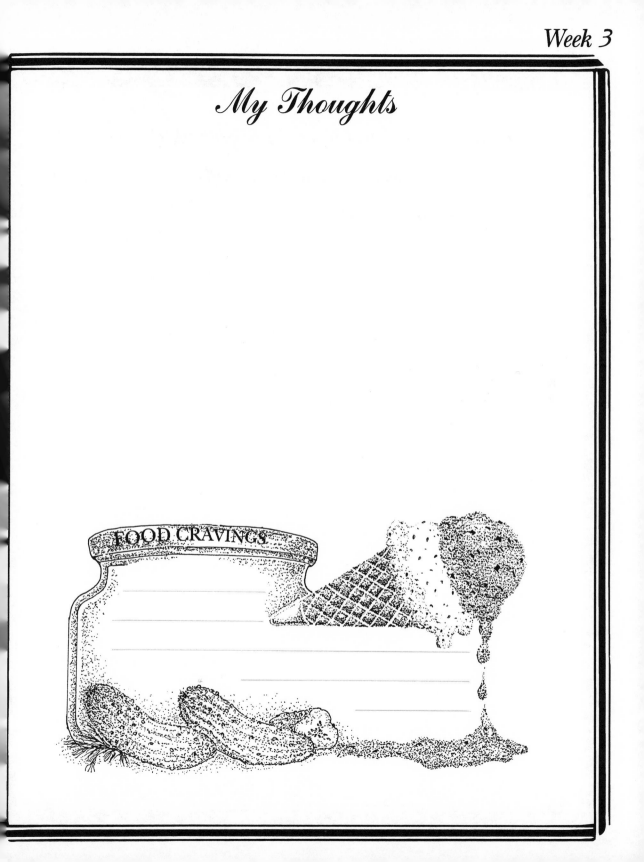

FOOD CRAVINGS

Is there anything I'm planning to give up during pregnancy, like smoking, drinking, caffeine or junk food? How do I feel about that?

My Dreams

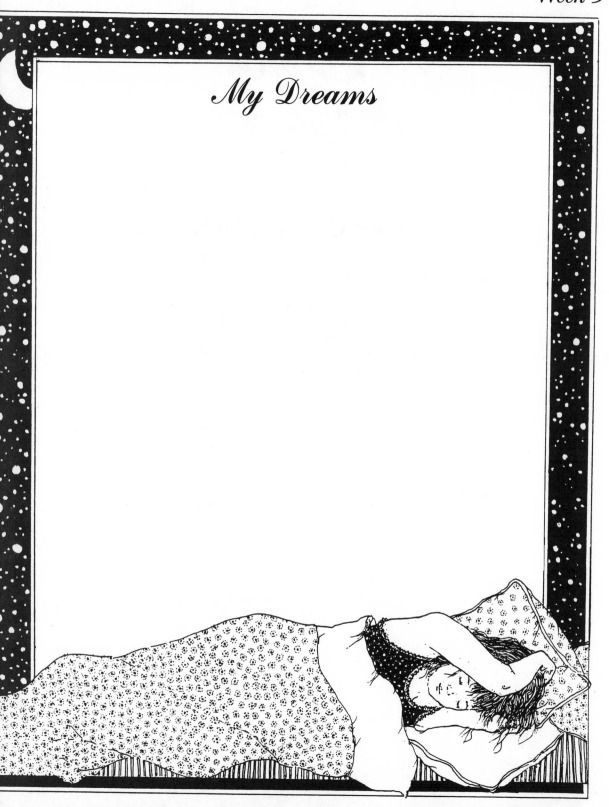

Your Growing Baby

During the fourth week the cells rapidly multiply into groups that will later become different structures.

By the end of the fourth week, the minuscule embryo has formed into the shape of a tadpole. The rudimentary beginnings of arms occur on the twenty- sixth day, and on the twenty-eighth day, the basic beginnings of legs, which will be slower in development than the arms.

The embryo is less than one-tenth of an inch long, or smaller than a grain of rice, and would be barely visible to your naked eye.

My Thoughts

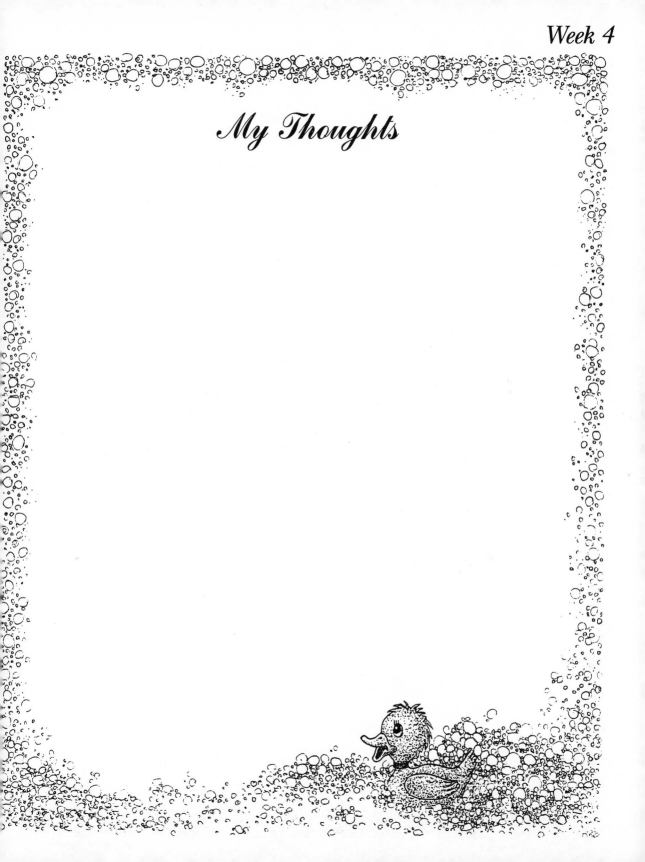

I've had a change in appetite, or food has affected me in some unusual ways . . .

My Dreams

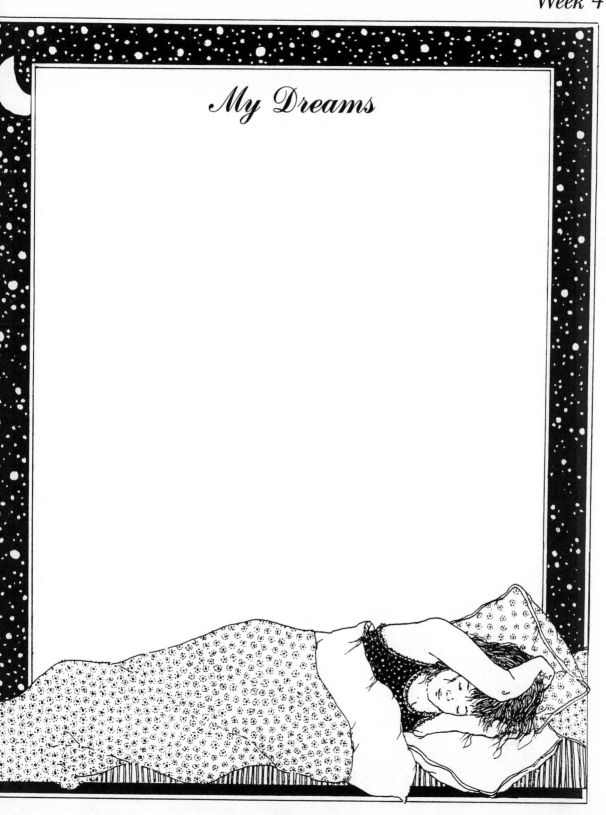

My First Doctor Visit

I am _____ weeks pregnant

My probable due date is _____

Weight _____ lbs.

How much more than my usual weight? _____ lbs.

Fundal height _____

Blood pressure _____

Urine (sugar, protein?) _____

Other tests? _____

Thigh measurement:

My (left/right) thigh is _____ inches.

My Disappearing Waist

My waist now is _____ inches, which is pretty much my

usual size (plus _____ inches).

Comments or Instructions from My Care Giver(s):

_____

_____

_____

_____

Questions I Want to Remember to Ask:

_____

_____

_____

_____

TUMMY PHOTO

My Thoughts on the Medical Care I'm Getting:

Your Growing Baby

By the end of the fifth week the foundation has been laid for what will be your baby's brain, spinal cord, and nervous system. Groups of tissue are developing that will later become your baby's spine, ribs, and abdominal muscles. Your baby's backbone is also forming, with five to eight vertebrae laid down.

The neural tube forms, which is the first step in the development of the central nervous system: one end of this will become your baby's brain, and other end the spinal cord.

A tubular, S-shaped heart is beginning to beat. This beating heart is located on the outside of the body, not yet inside the chest cavity.

The developing baby is only a fraction of an inch long.

My Thoughts

OLD WIVES' TALES AND ADVICE

*A pregnant woman is not allowed to wash clothes in the river,
because her presence will drive away the fish.*

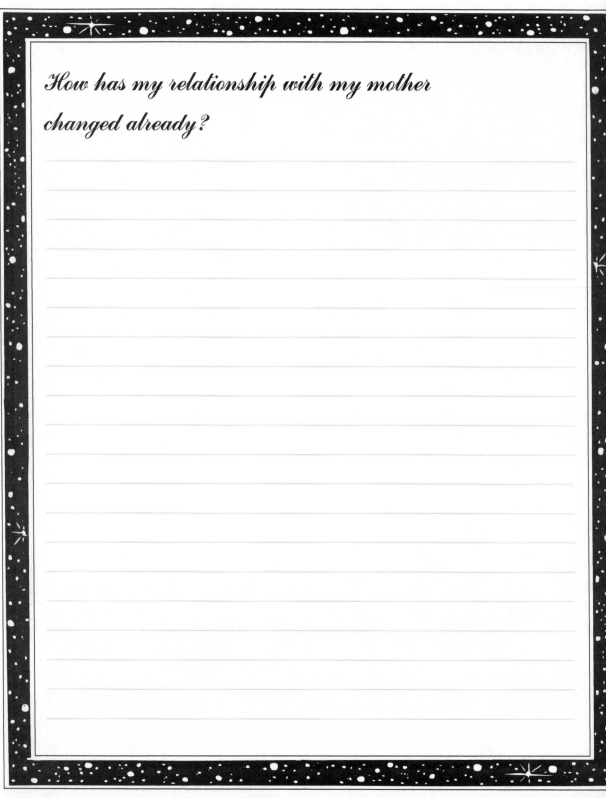

How has my relationship with my mother changed already?

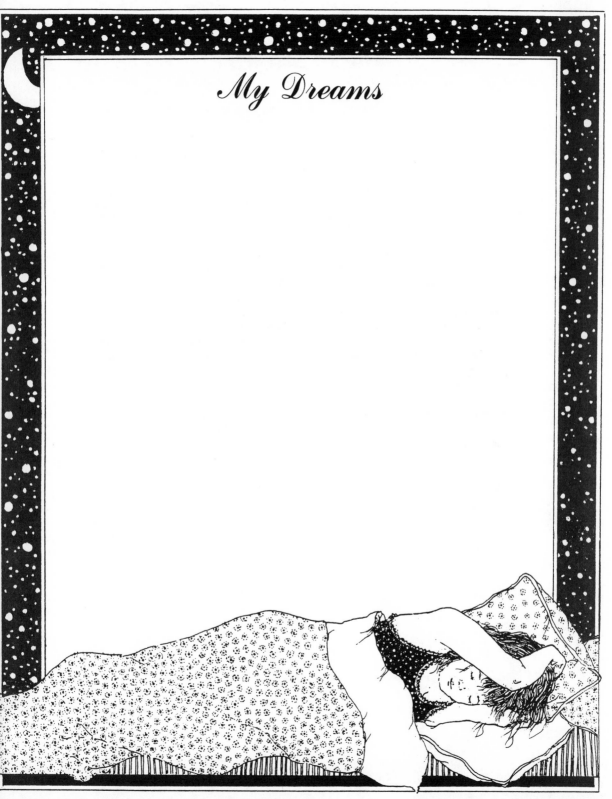

My Dreams

Your Growing Baby

At the beginning of the sixth week the head is starting to form, with the beginning of a brain. There are depressions beneath the skin where the eyes and ears will later appear.

A two-chamber heart is forming, which will, of course, eventually be a four-chamber organ. The baby's intestinal tract is forming, which starts from the mouth cavity downward, although the mouth cannot yet open.

The stalk connecting the embryo to the placenta begins to grow into the umbilical cord, with blood vessels inside it through which you will nourish your growing child.

There is quite a long rudimentary tail, which is an extension of the spinal column. By the end of this week all the backbone has been laid down and the spinal canal is closed over, although the lower part of the back is still undeveloped. The baby grows in a curved seahorse shape because the blocks of tissue in the back of the embryo grow more quickly than those in front.

At the corners of the body there are tiny limb buds (which first appeared in the fourth week), which will later become the arms and legs.

The germ cells have appeared, which will later become either ovaries or testes.

By the end of this week your baby will be one-fourth inch long.

My Thoughts

Names and Nicknames

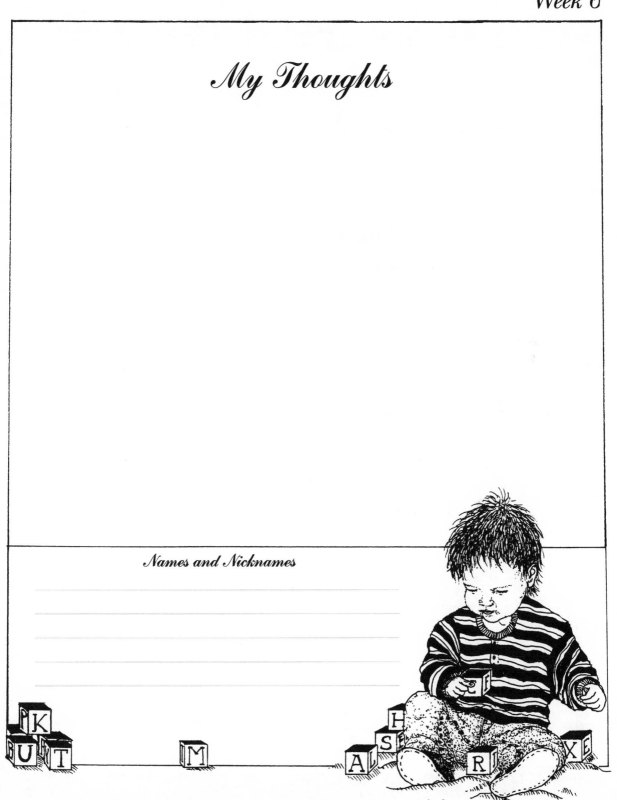

Have I had moments of feeling ambivalent about being pregnant? Had doubts about whether this is the right time in my life to have a child?

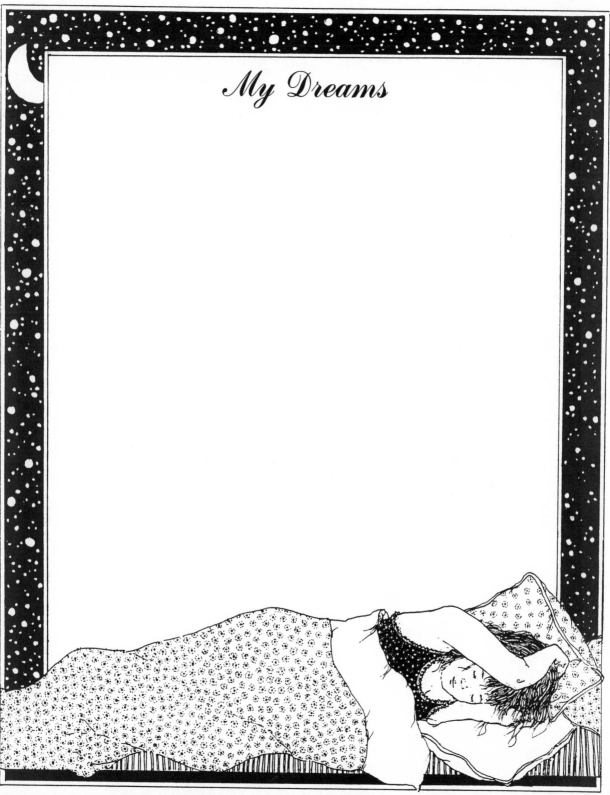

My Dreams

Your Growing Baby

Nerve and muscle work together for the first time now. The baby has reflexes and makes spontaneous movements, although you probably won't feel these until the sixteenth to twenty-sixth weeks.

The chest and abdomen are completely formed: the lung buds are appearing, and the heart is now inside the body. The heart is still a simple structure, but it has developed four chambers, beating with enough strength to circulate blood cells through the blood vessels.

By the end of this week your baby's brain and spinal cord will be almost complete. During this week the embryo becomes a primitive small-scale baby, less than one inch long, with a lumpy head that is bent forward on the chest. The baby's mouth can open, with lips and a tongue visible. The face looks more human, with eyes perceptible through closed lids, and openings for the nostrils.

Shell-like external ears are developing, although they don't yet protrude. This is an important week for the growth of your baby's inner ear: the middle part of the ear develops, which is responsible for balance as well as hearing.

The limb buds are growing rapidly, and there is a paddle shape to what will be arms and legs. The hands have the beginning of fingers and thumbs; the toes are stubby, but the big toes have appeared. The baby's arms are as long as a printed exclamation point(!).

The overall length is about one-half inch by the end of the seventh week, or roughly the size of your thumbnail.

My Thoughts

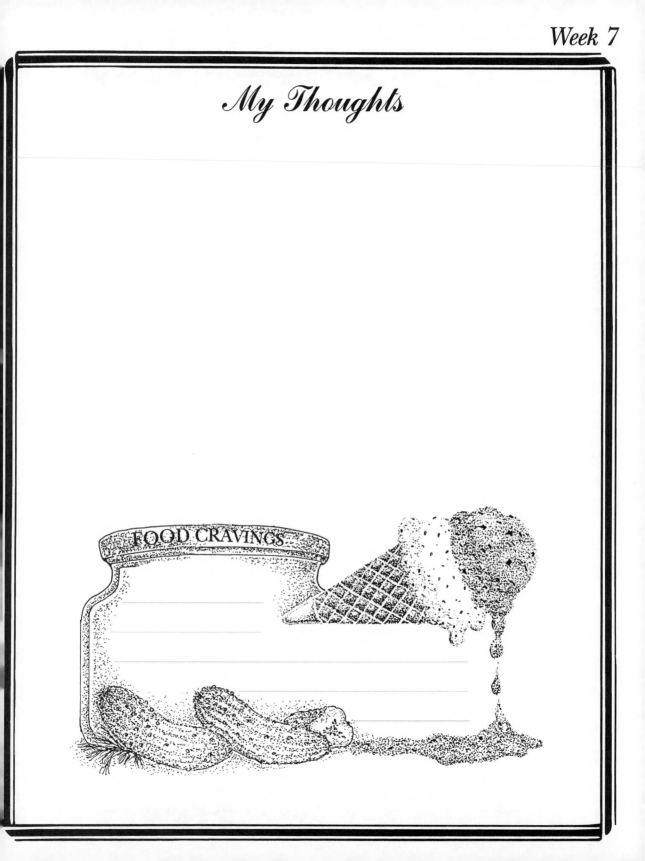

FOOD CRAVINGS

How have my parents and in-laws reacted to my pregnancy? And what kind of grandparents do I imagine they will make?

My Dreams

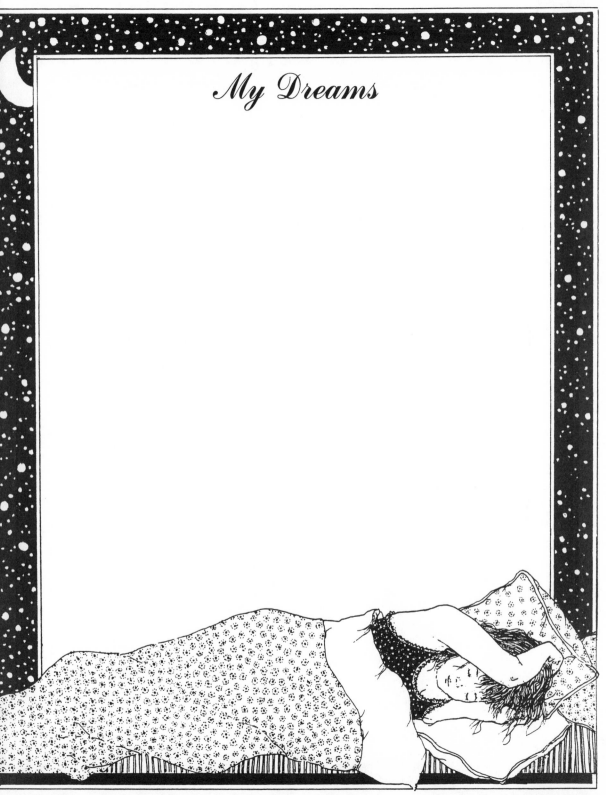

Week 8
(End of Second Month)

Your Growing Baby

In this week, actually on the forty-seventh day of your pregnancy, the first true bone cells begin to replace cartilage. This is the baby's official transition from embryo to fetus. The bones of her arms and legs start to harden and elongate. Critical joints like the knees, hips, shoulders, and elbows are forming. Her toes and fingers are more pronounced, although they are joined by webs of skin. By the end of this week the baby's physical structure is complete, with a skeleton made of cartilage, which will gradually be replaced by bone cells. However, her body has a fishlike shape, and her head is disproportionately large. Her face and jaw are fully formed, with the teeth and facial muscles still developing. Her eyes are covered by skin that will eventually split to form the eyelids.

Her heart is now pumping forcefully with a regular rhythm. Blood vessels are visible through her transparent skin.

All the major organs—heart, brain, lungs, kidneys, liver, and intestine—are in place, although not yet fully developed. The clitoris or penis begins to appear, and the ovaries or testicles are taking form, although at this point you could not tell just by looking whether it's a girl or boy.

By the end of this second month the baby weighs about one-third of an ounce (less than an aspirin tablet) and is a little more than one inch long.

My Thoughts

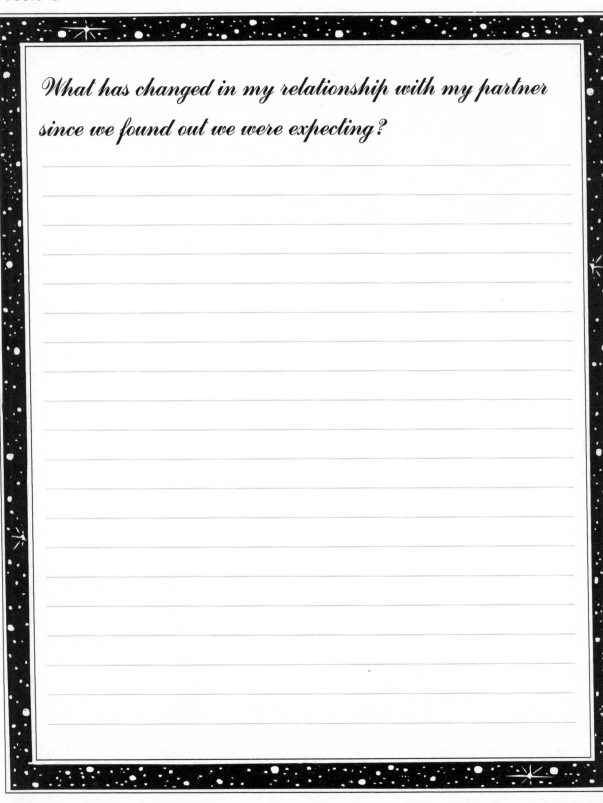

What has changed in my relationship with my partner since we found out we were expecting?

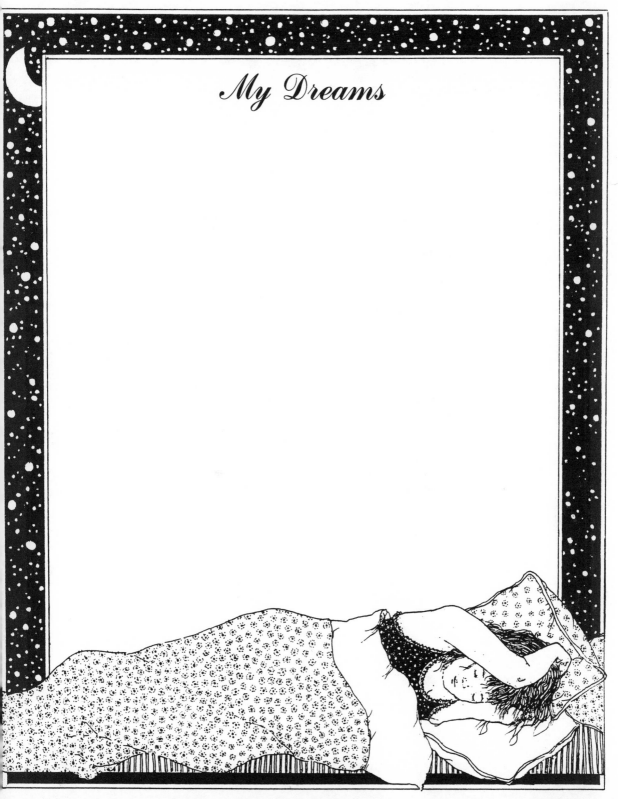

My Dreams

Your Growing Baby

Physical refinements are taking place and the baby's face is becoming quite human, except for the jaws, which aren't fully developed. During these seven days the baby will start to open her mouth; once the upper and lower jaws fuse at the sides, she'll be able to suck and chew. The palate to form the roof of the mouth is closing. Taste buds (the glands that produce saliva) appear, and the vocal cords are developing. Tooth buds for the baby teeth are present. Her eyes, which were at the sides of her head, are moving to the front, and their development is complete, although they still have a membrane eyelid. A nose has appeared.

The fastest growth this week is in the limbs, hands, and feet: fingers and toes are becoming defined, and nail beds are forming for eventual nails.

The chest cavity becomes separated from the abdominal cavity by a band of muscle that will later develop into the diaphragm, a muscle that plays an important part in breathing. The heart has completed forming four chambers and is beating 117 to 157 beats per minute.

The baby is just over an inch in length this week; her hands are now about as big (one-fourth inch) as the whole embryo was a month ago.

Getting to Know My Baby

Since it's a bit soon for my baby to be able to let me know anything about himself yet, these are the qualities and attributes that I hope my child will have . . .

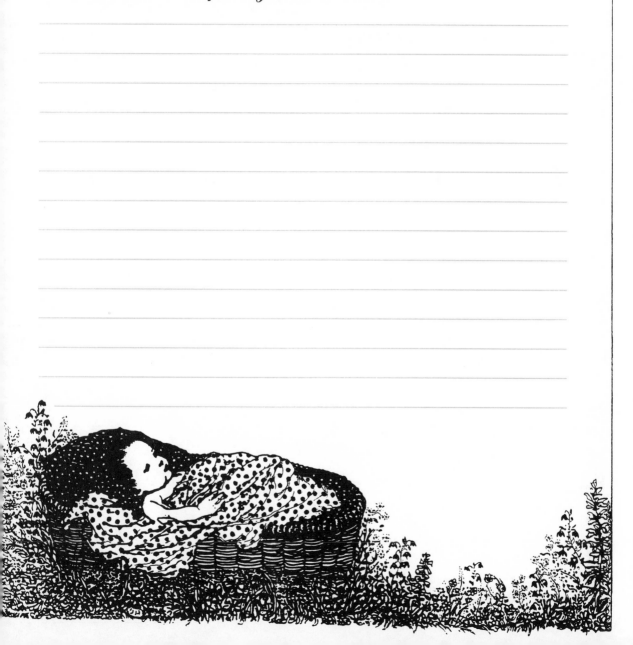

If I have a job, what thoughts have I had about continuing my work after the baby is born? If I don't have a job, in what ways do I imagine my daily life will change once the baby is born?

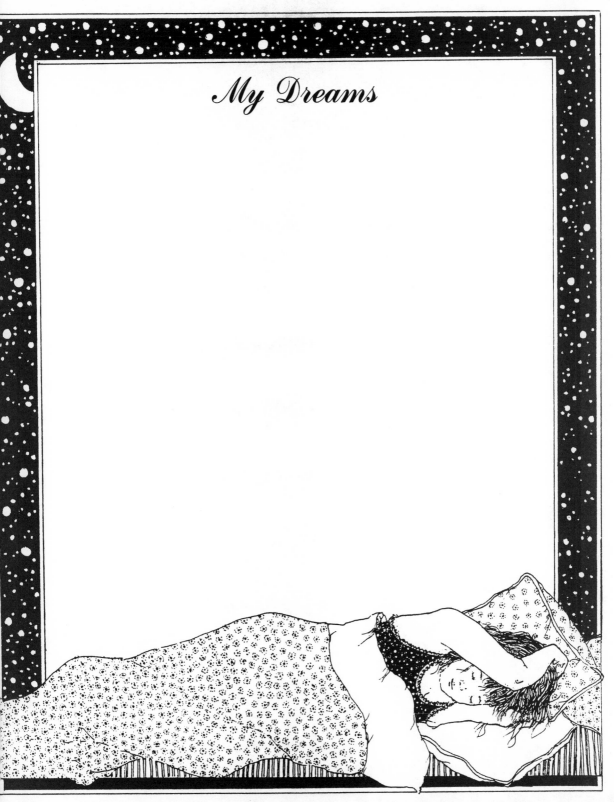

My Dreams

Your Growing Baby

The baby's brain has developed quickly in the past month so that his head is still large in proportion to his body. This week marks the final development of the ears: the inner portion is complete, and the external parts are beginning to grow.

The stomach and intestines have formed in the abdomen, and the muscle wall of the intestinal tract is developing.

The kidneys are moving into their permanent positions and will have developed by the end of this month.

The lungs are growing inside the chest cavity.

The major blood vessels are assuming their final form. The umbilical cord has fully formed, and blood is circulating through it.

By this week the baby has grown to just under one and a half inches.

My Thoughts

OLD WIVES' TALES AND ADVICE

If a pregnant woman hears an owl hooting, it's a sign she'll have a girl.
If the bridge in her nose spreads, she'll have a boy.

What doubts, dreams, and hopes do I have about the new life ahead of me?

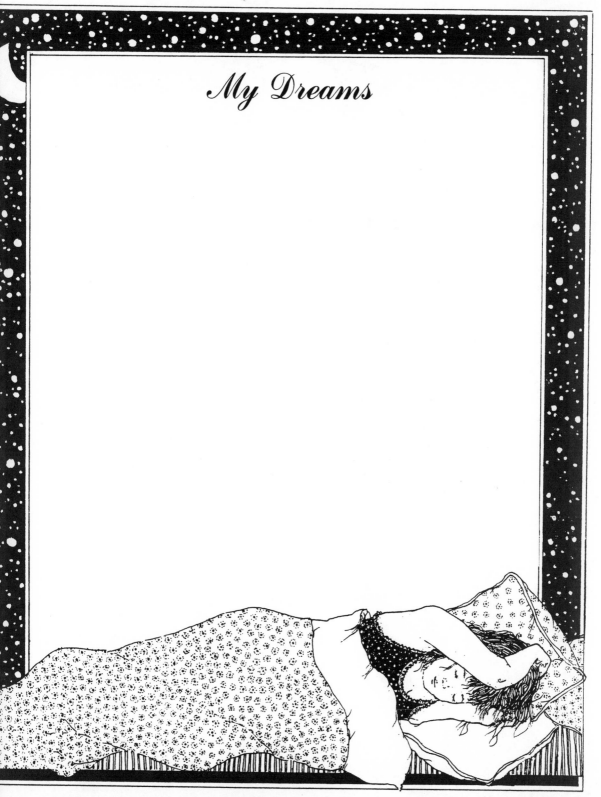

My Dreams

Your Growing Baby

At eleven weeks the baby is now able to swallow, and the cycle of circulation starts. The kidneys have formed, and the urinary system is operating: the baby swallows amniotic fluid and urinates it back into the amniotic fluid in which he floats.

All your baby's essential organs will have formed by the end of this week, and most of them are beginning to function. From this point forward, these internal organs will simply continue to grow. The liver, for example, is now producing bile. Your baby's heart is pumping blood to all parts of his body, and is also pumping blood through the umbilical cord to what is going to become the placenta.

Your baby is now clearly recognizable as a tiny human, with a face that's becoming more rounded. The back of his head has enlarged, which puts his eyes in a more natural position than before; his ears have a flatter shape and are continuing to develop. His limbs are still short and skinny, but his ankles and wrists have formed, and his elbows and knees are taking shape. His toes and fingers are now clearly separated and developed.

The baby's length is now approximately two inches.

My Thoughts

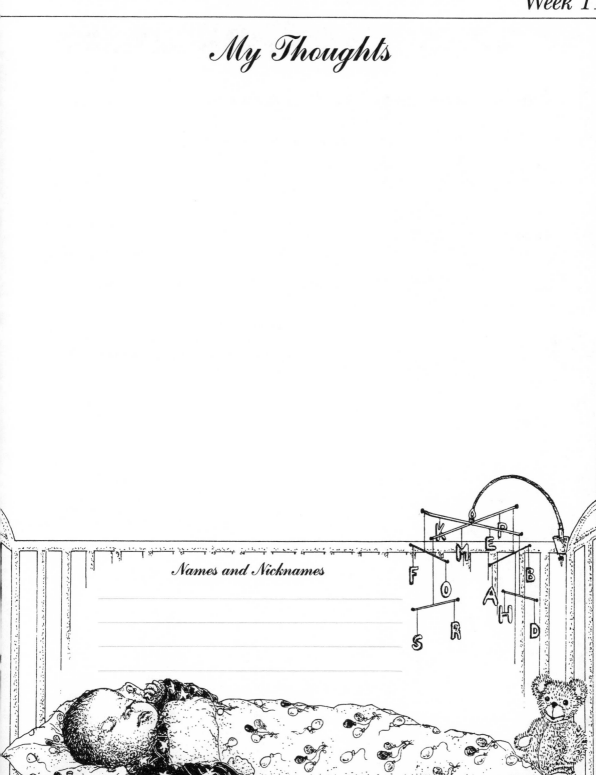

Names and Nicknames

What are some ways in which being pregnant has given me physical problems such as nausea, difficulty sleeping, or leg cramps?

My Dreams

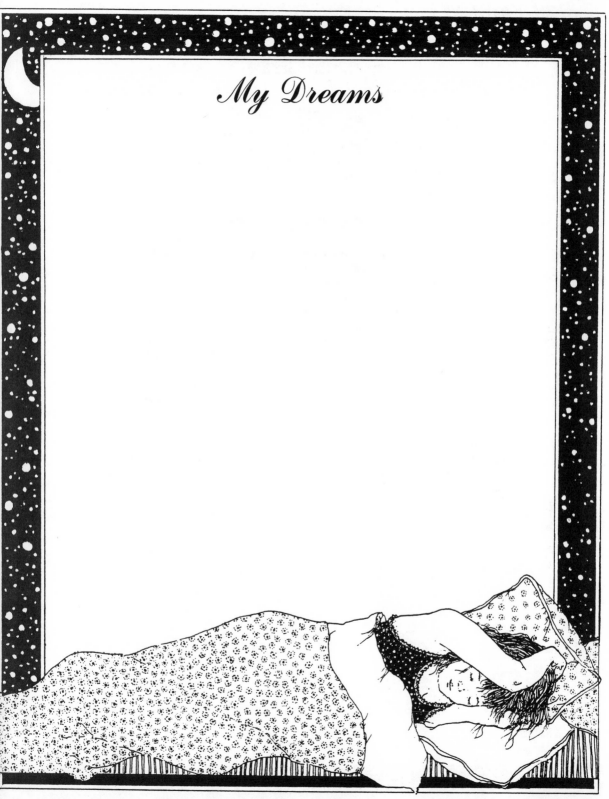

Week 12
(End of Third Month)

Your Growing Baby

When the brain signals, the baby's muscles now respond and she kicks. However, all movements reflex from the spinal cord since the brain is not yet sufficiently organized to control them (and it won't be until after birth). The baby is becoming active, but unless you are very slender, it is rare to feel the movement yet. She can make stepping movements and even curl her toes. Her brain and muscles coordinate so that her arms bend and can rotate at the wrist and elbow; her fingers close so that she can form a tight fist or unclench it.

Her ears are completely formed; she can make facial expressions like pressing her lips together and frowning.

She is already using the muscles required for breathing after birth.

The female external vulva and the male penis have gradually been molded during the second and third months. The male scrotum appears during the twelfth week, although it is still difficult to distinguish the baby's sex at this point.

This week the umbilical cord starts to circulate blood between the baby and the group of membranes attached to the wall of your uterus. Your baby's body has begun to depend on these membranes for nourishment; the placenta begins to function this week.

By the end of the third month the baby weighs a little more than one-half ounce.

My Thoughts

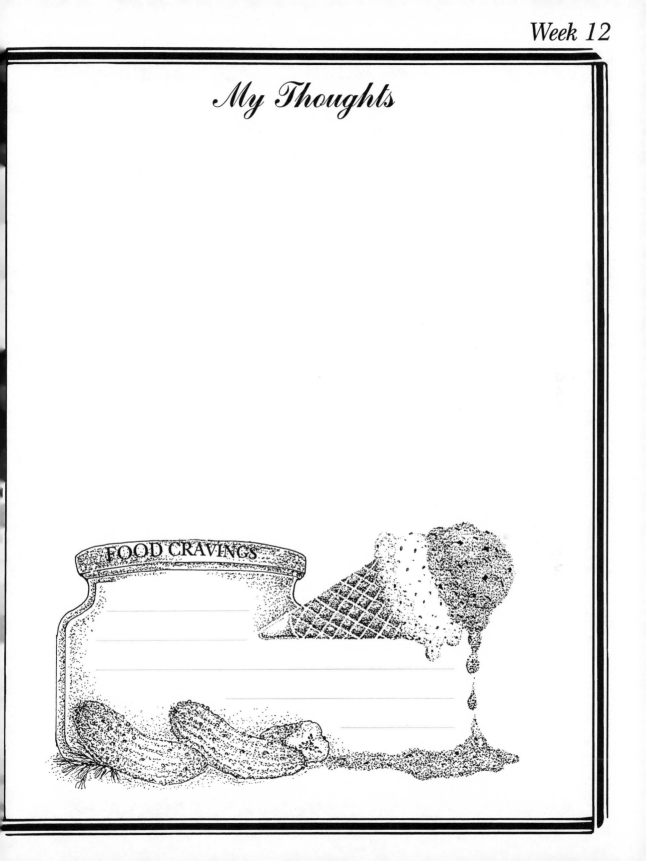

FOOD CRAVINGS

Do I wonder whether I'll be a good mother? What doubts do I have about myself as a mom?

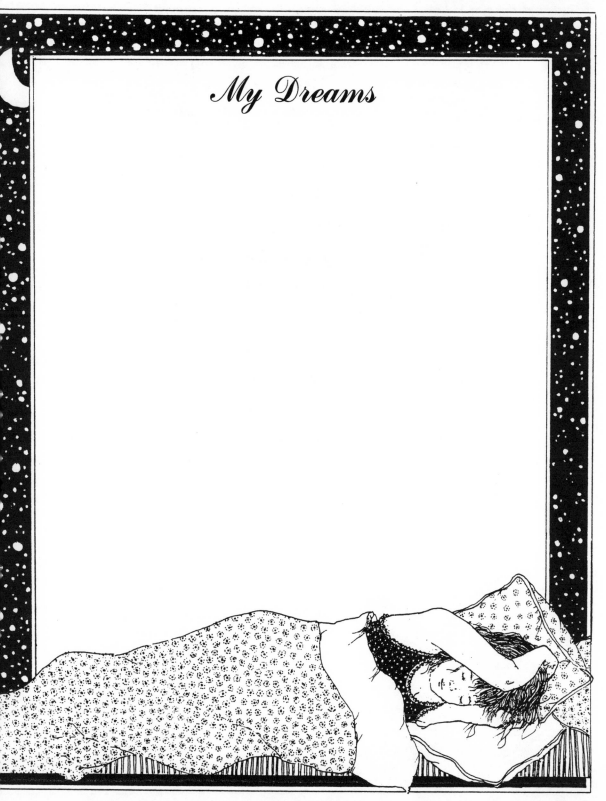

My Dreams

My Third-Month (12 Week) Doctor Visit

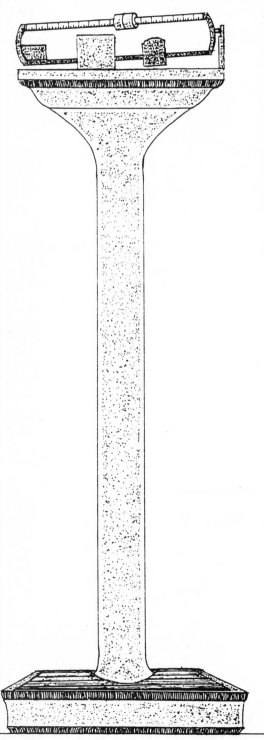

Weight _____ lbs.

Pounds gained since last visit _____ lbs.

Fundal height _____

Blood pressure _____

Urine (sugar, protein?) _____

Other tests? _____

Thigh measurement:

My (left/right) thigh is _____ inches (_____ inches more than the last time I measured.)

My Disappearing Waist

My gradually disappearing waist is _____ inches (_____ inches more than the last time I checked).

Comments or Instructions from My Care Giver(s):

_____

_____

_____

_____

_____

Questions I Want to Remember to Ask:

_____

_____

_____

_____

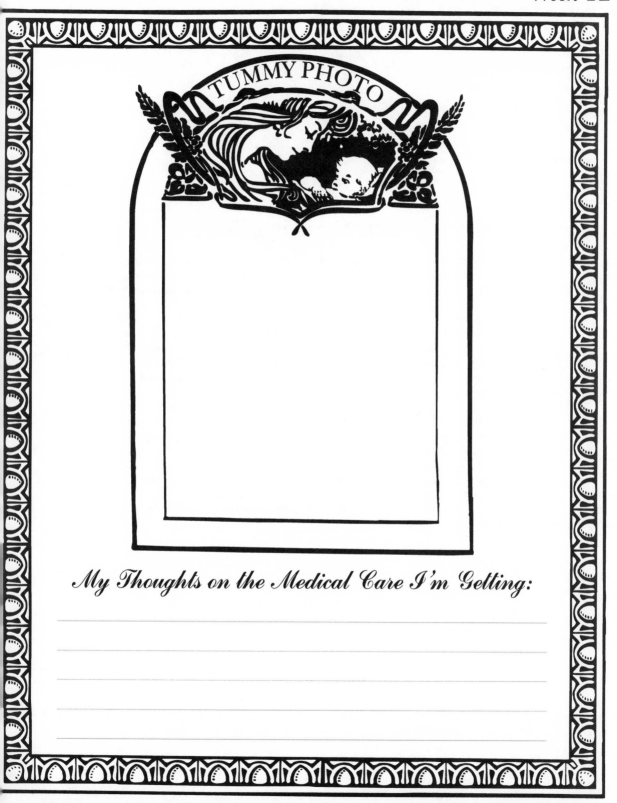

TUMMY PHOTO

My Thoughts on the Medical Care I'm Getting:

Your Growing Baby

By the end of this week your baby fills the uterine cavity and is now properly formed. His neck is now fully developed, allowing his head to move freely on his body. His face is formed, with the mouth, nose, and external ears completely developed.

A WORD ABOUT THE PLACENTA. The placenta is an organ created by your body to nourish your baby and excrete his waste products. The placenta looks like a large, roundish liver, an inch thick and measuring about eight inches in diameter. It was fully formed by last week and will be fully operational by next week. The placenta is attached on one side to your uterus and on the other side to the baby's umbilical cord. It is the baby's lifeline to you: your blood, carrying oxygen and nutrients, reaches the baby through a fine membrane into the placenta. The placenta functions like a sieve, passing oxygen, food, and protective antibodies from you to your baby (although harmful elements can also filter through). The baby gets rid of his waste products by filtering them through the placenta into your bloodstream, allowing you to excrete them. The blood from which the baby has already taken oxygen comes back through an artery in the umbilical cord into the placenta.

By the end of this week your baby is three inches long and weighs about one ounce.

Getting to Know My Baby

My baby seems to be aware of . . .

_____

_____

_____

_____

_____

_____

_____

My baby seems to respond to . . .

_____

_____

_____

_____

_____

_____

_____

How has my relationship changed with my mother and
mother-in-law since I got pregnant?

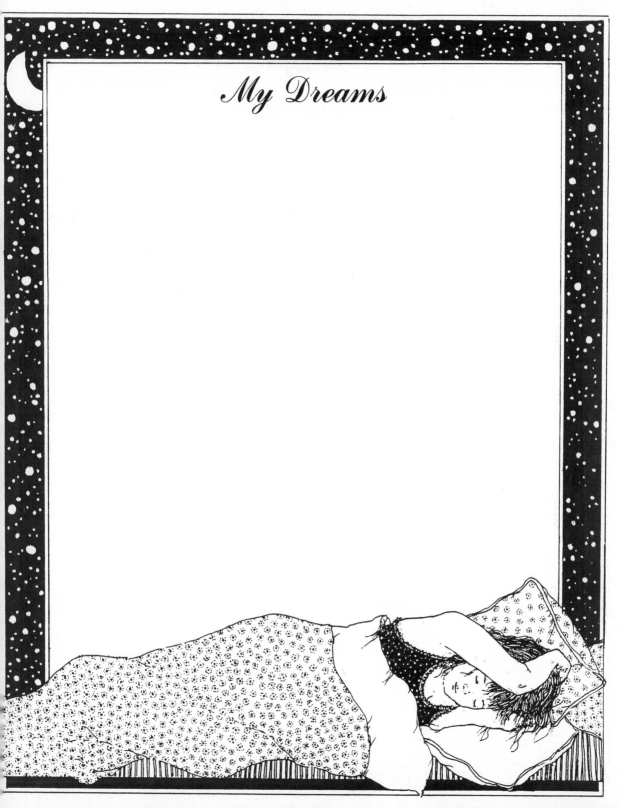

My Dreams

Your Growing Baby

This week marks the beginning of the second trimester of your pregnancy, the time when your baby does most of her growing and when her organs mature. The baby's heart is beating strongly (her heartbeat is almost twice as fast as yours), and you may be able to hear it in the doctor's office.

Her nervous system has begun to function, and her muscles respond to stimulation from her brain. Her arms continue their development of specialized functions and can grasp, curl, and make fists. Her movements are more vigorous, but you probably don't feel them yet. The baby develops her muscles by exercising energetically inside you, which she does with ease, floating in the amniotic fluid.

During this past week your baby more than doubled in weight. She now weighs over two ounces and measures around four inches in length.

My Thoughts

OLD WIVES' TALES AND ADVICE

If you are "big in the front" early in your pregnancy, expect a baby boy.
If you grow "big in the back," you'll give birth to a girl.

In what ways has my partner changed during my pregnancy?

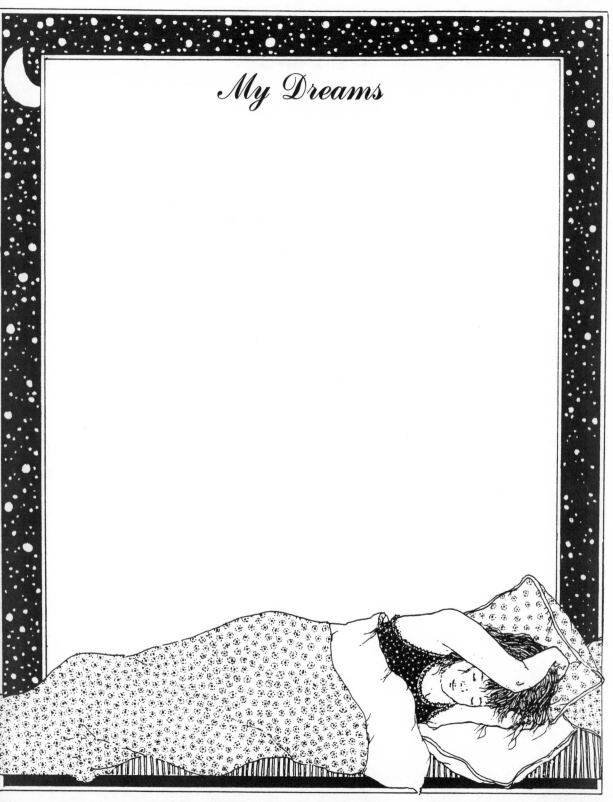

My Dreams

Your Growing Baby

Your baby is probably able to hear by now, because the three tiny bones of his middle ear are the first of his bones to harden. From now on you are what he will be listening to! Liquid is a good sound conductor, so through the amniotic fluid the baby can hear your heart beating, your stomach rumbling, and the sound of your voice. Certain sounds from outside the womb can also reach him. However, his brain is not yet sufficiently developed to process the information: the auditory centers in the brain (which decipher the sounds received) have not yet fully formed.

Your baby has begun to grow hair sometime in the past week: by now there's a little fluff on his head, and he has eyebrows along with white eyelashes. In addition, the *lanugo* starts to grow: a fine, downy hair begins to appear all over your baby's face and body, which keeps his temperature constant. Most of this hair will disappear before he is born; whatever is left will fall out soon after birth.

The baby now measures somewhat more than five inches and weighs roughly three and a half ounces.

My Thoughts

Names and Nicknames

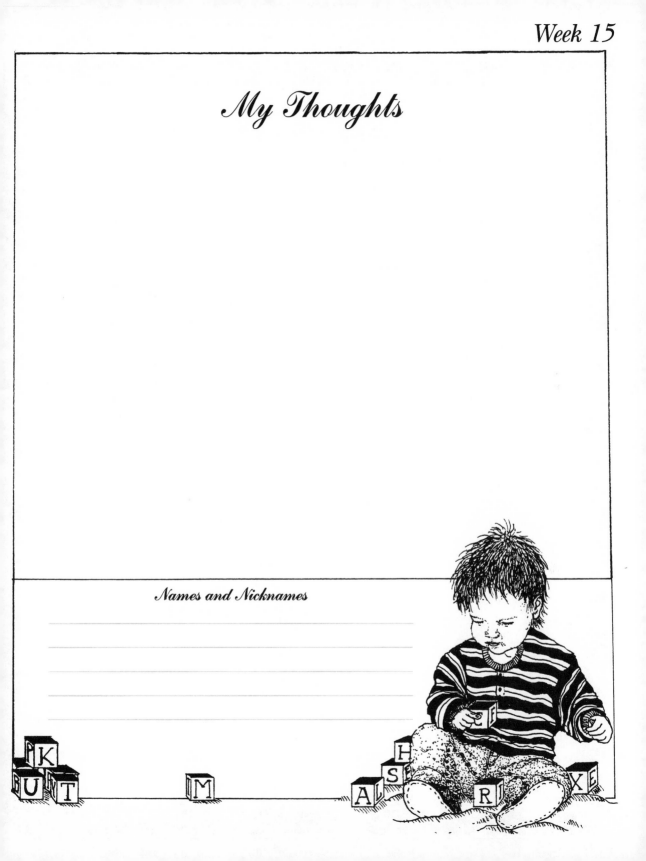

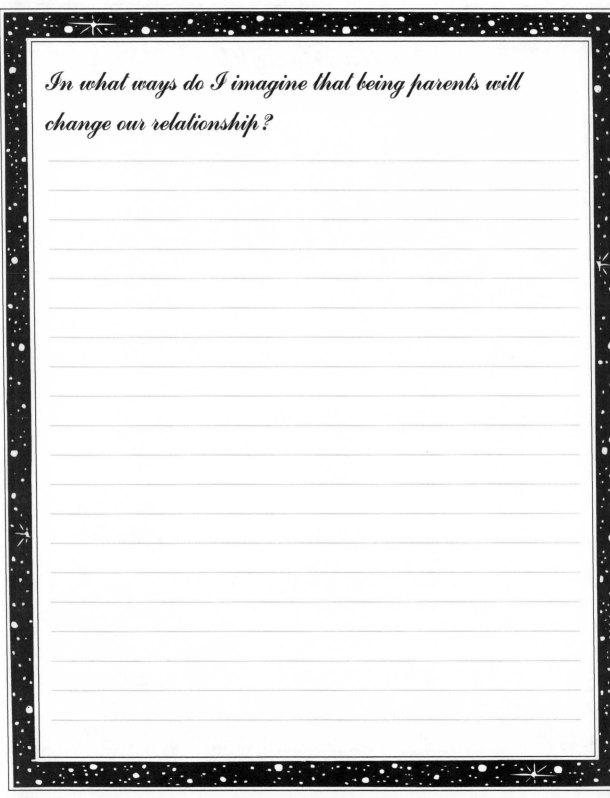

In what ways do I imagine that being parents will change our relationship?

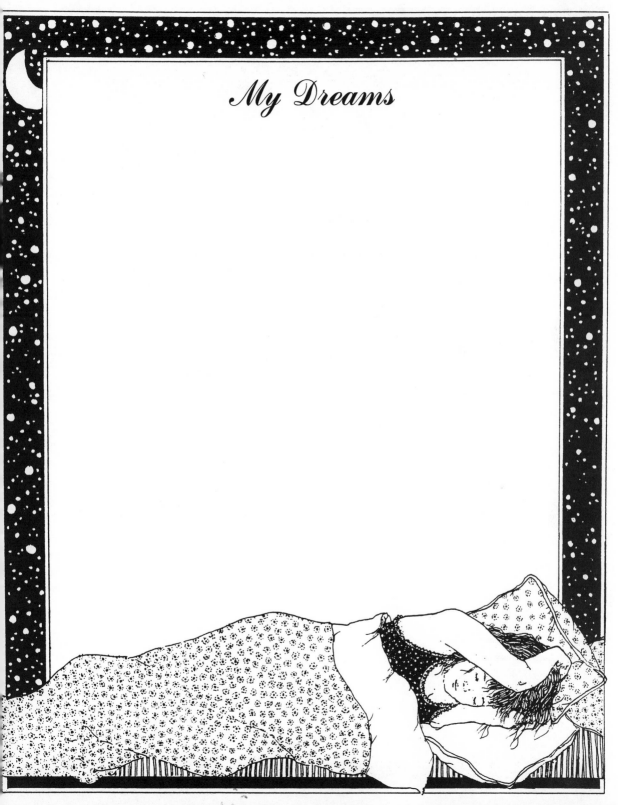

My Dreams

Your Growing Baby

By the end of the fourth month the baby will suck if her lips are stroked. If a bitter substance like iodine is introduced into the amniotic fluid, she will grimace and stop swallowing; if a sweetener is introduced, she usually drinks twice as quickly. If a bright light is shined on your abdomen, the baby will gradually move her hands up to shield her eyes.

In these weeks the baby is moving actively and can even turn somersaults, although if this is your first child, you probably won't feel these movements yet.

At sixteen weeks some babies may begin to suck their thumb, which helps develop coordination and has a soothing effect. At this point, your baby can yawn, stretch, and make facial expressions. She can also swallow and may get hiccups.

Her eyes are large, spaced wide apart, and closed.

During the fourth month the baby grows so much, she quadruples her weight and doubles her height of the third month. She now weighs about seven ounces and is six inches long.

My Thoughts

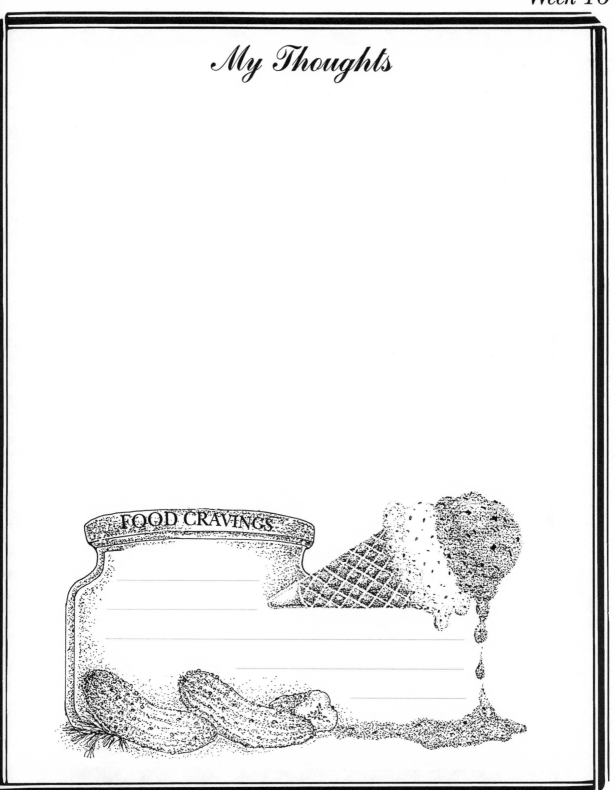

FOOD CRAVINGS

How have I told my other children or stepchildren about the new baby? What was their reaction?

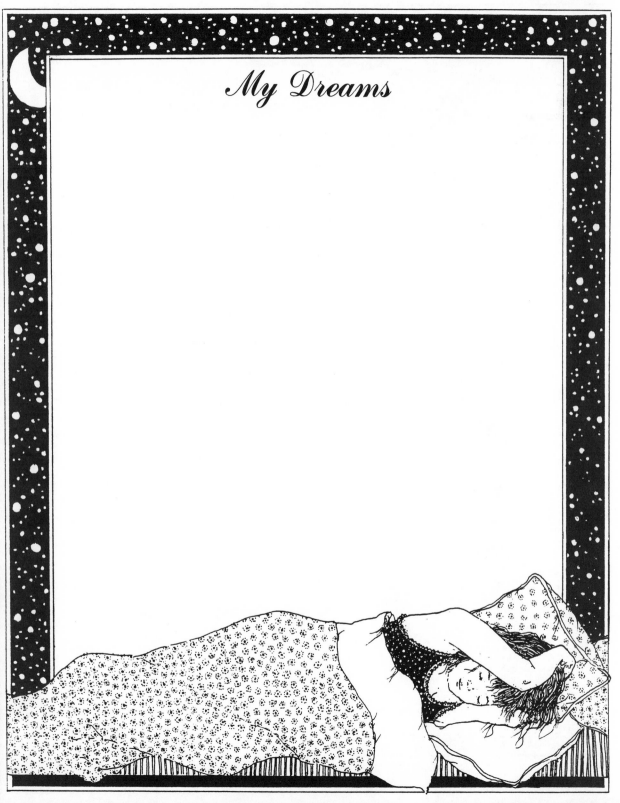

My Dreams

My Fourth-Month (16 Week) Doctor Visit

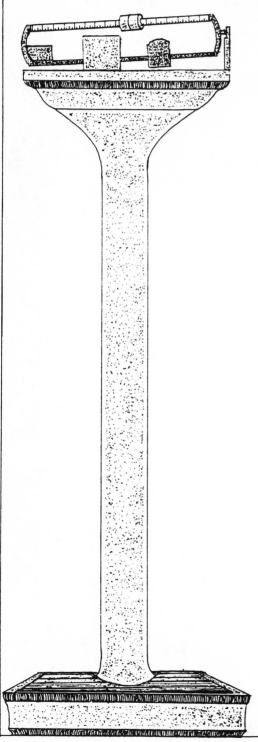

Weight _____ lbs.

Pounds gained since last visit _____ lbs.

Fundal height _____

Blood pressure _____

Urine (sugar, protein?) _____

Other tests? _____

Thigh measurement:

My (left/right) thigh is _____ inches

(_____ inches more than last month).

My Disappearing Waist

My disappearing waist is _____ inches

(_____ inches more than last month).

Comments or Instructions from My Care Giver(s):

_____

_____

_____

_____

_____

Questions I Want to Remember to Ask:

_____

_____

_____

_____

_____

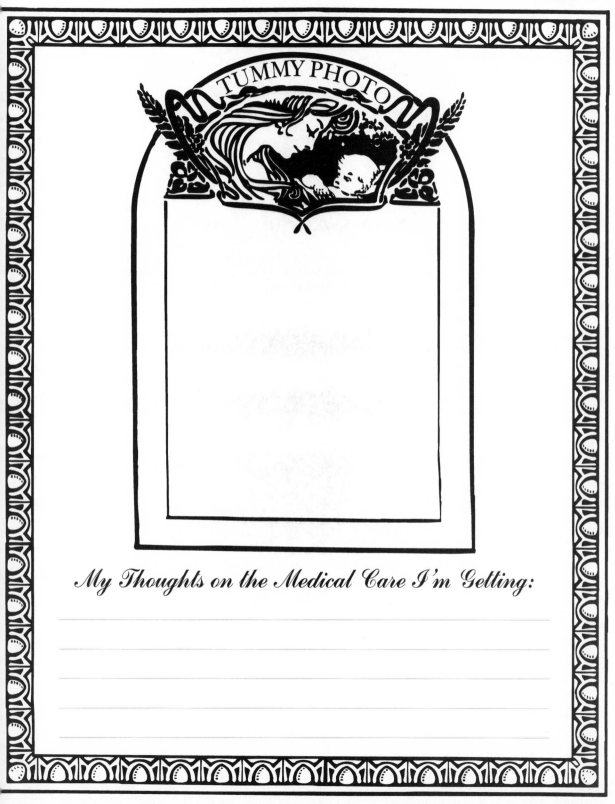

TUMMY PHOTO

My Thoughts on the Medical Care I'm Getting:

Your Growing Baby

Your baby's skin is developing and is transparent, appearing red because the blood vessels are visible through it. The baby's skin has begun to develop *vernix,* a white protective coating like cream cheese. The *lanugo* (the fine hair all over the baby's body) can make wavelike patterns on the baby's skin because she is immersed in liquid.

The hair on her head, eyebrows, and eyelashes is filling out.

Hard nails form on the nail beds, with the toenails developing a bit later than fingernails.

Both sexes develop nipples and underlying mammary glands. The external genital organs have now developed sufficiently for your baby's sex to be detected by ultrasound.

Your baby measures a little more than seven inches in length and now weighs more than the placenta does.

Getting to Know My Baby

Does my baby react yet to any particular foods that I eat?

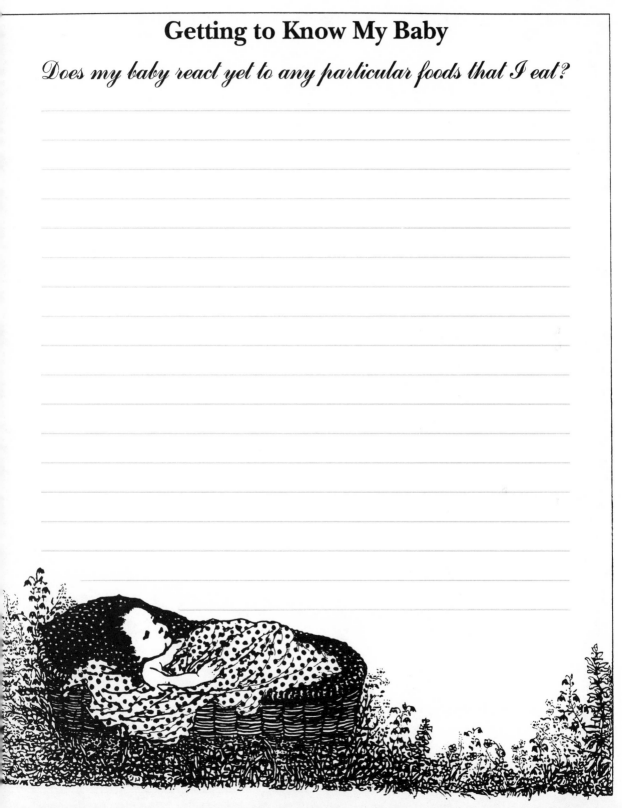

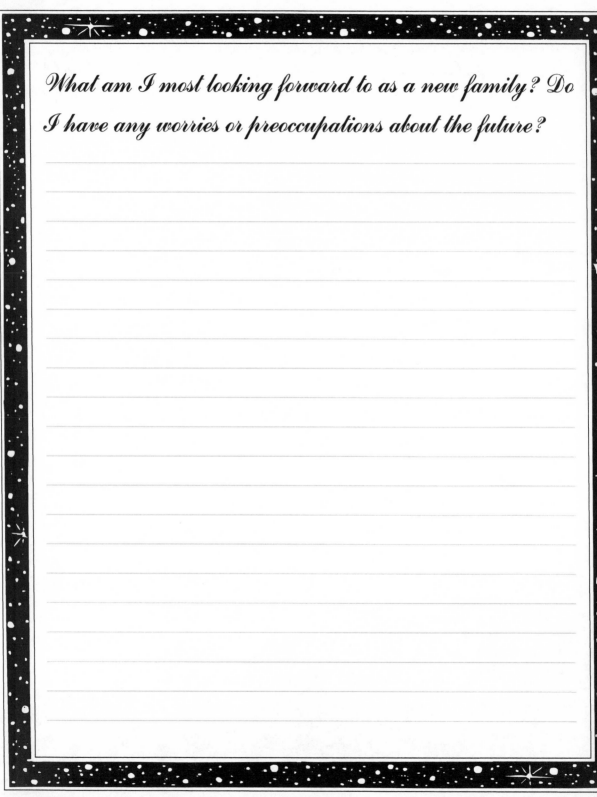

What am I most looking forward to as a new family? Do I have any worries or preoccupations about the future?

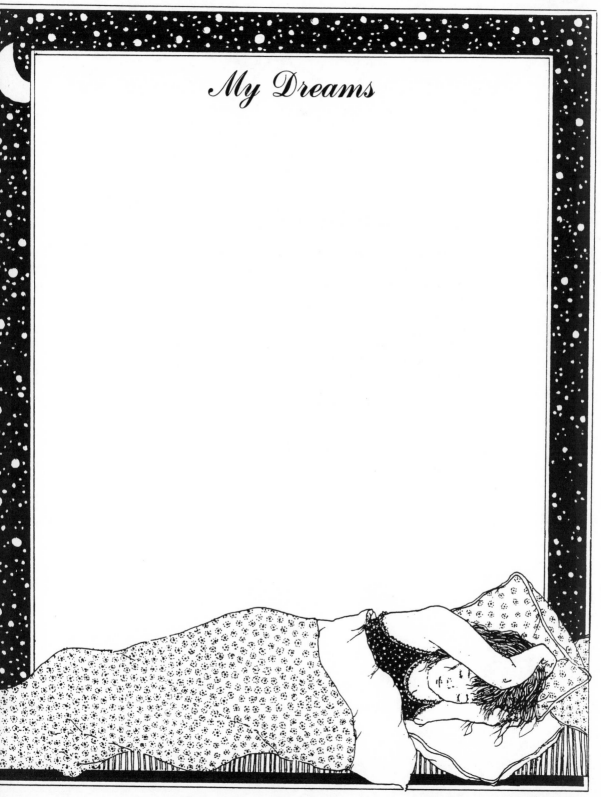

My Dreams

Your Growing Baby

The baby can now hear sounds outside your body; if a loud sound is made next to you, the unborn baby will raise his hands and cover his ears. Very loud sounds have been known to startle a baby enough to make him jump inside you.

His limbs are fully developed, and all his joints are able to move, so he's testing his reflexes, kicking and punching with well-formed arms and legs. He is moving around much of the time, and it's during this week that you may feel his gyrations for the first time. He can twist, turn, and wiggle inside you—and may practice when you least expect it! The baby's muscles are now almost fully developed, including the muscles in his chest, which are beginning to make movements similar to those that he will use for respiration later on.

Tiny air sacs, known as *alveoli,* which he'll need later in order to breathe, are forming inside his developing lungs.

Your baby measures about eight inches long this week.

My Thoughts

OLD WIVES' TALES AND ADVICE

*If a pregnant woman handles flowers too much,
her baby will have a poor sense of smell.*

How is being pregnant different from my expectations?

My Dreams

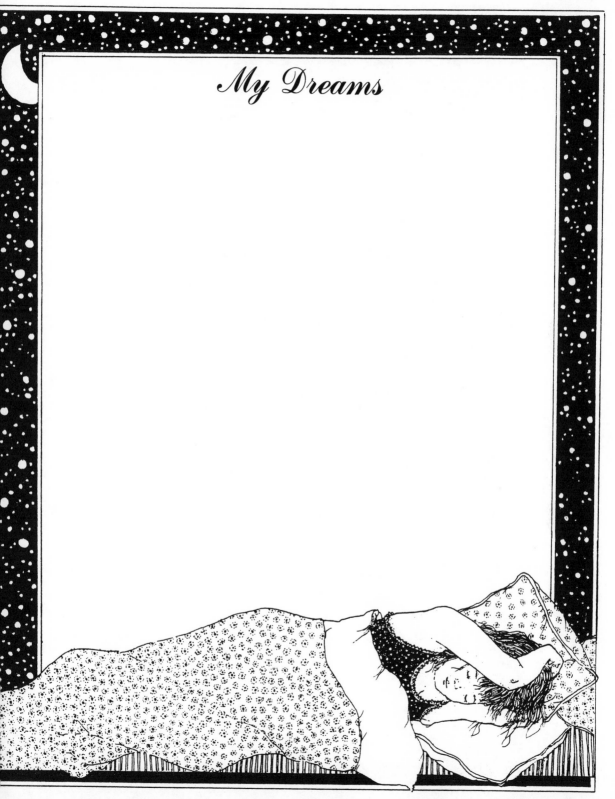

Your Growing Baby

If you haven't felt the baby yet, you'll probably perceive the baby's movements this week.

This week buds for permanent teeth begin forming behind those that have already developed for her baby teeth.

In some babies, it is only during this week that they begin to grow hair and eyebrows, and white eyelashes appear.

The amniotic fluid is filled with salts and other nutrients that the baby absorbs through her skin, as she has been doing throughout your pregnancy. This fluid is always fresh because it's constantly being produced by your body and is completely replenished every six hours. At this stage in development your baby is drinking quite a lot of amniotic fluid; her stomach begins to secrete gastric juices, enabling her body to absorb those liquids. After the fluid is absorbed, her kidneys filter the fluid and excrete it back into the amniotic sac.

Your baby now measures about nine inches long.

My Thoughts

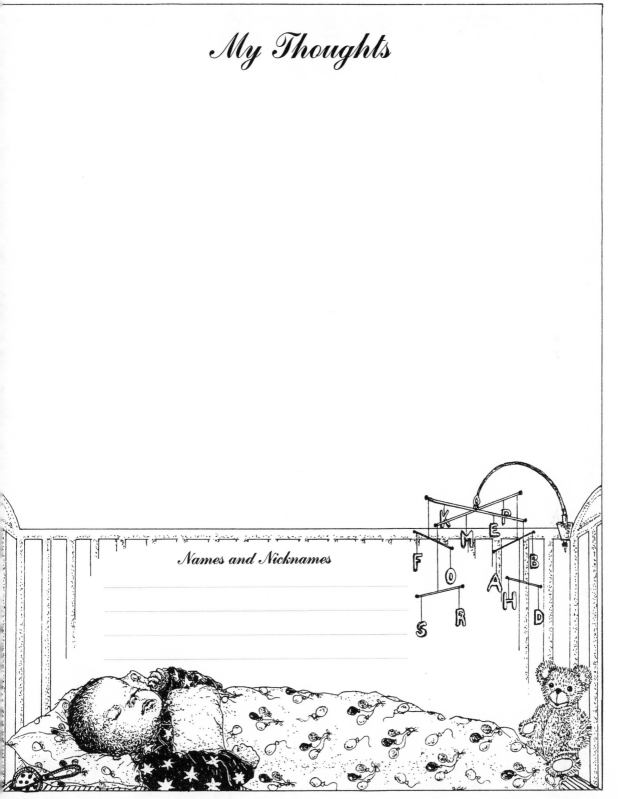

Names and Nicknames

What were my feelings when I first felt the baby move?

My Dreams

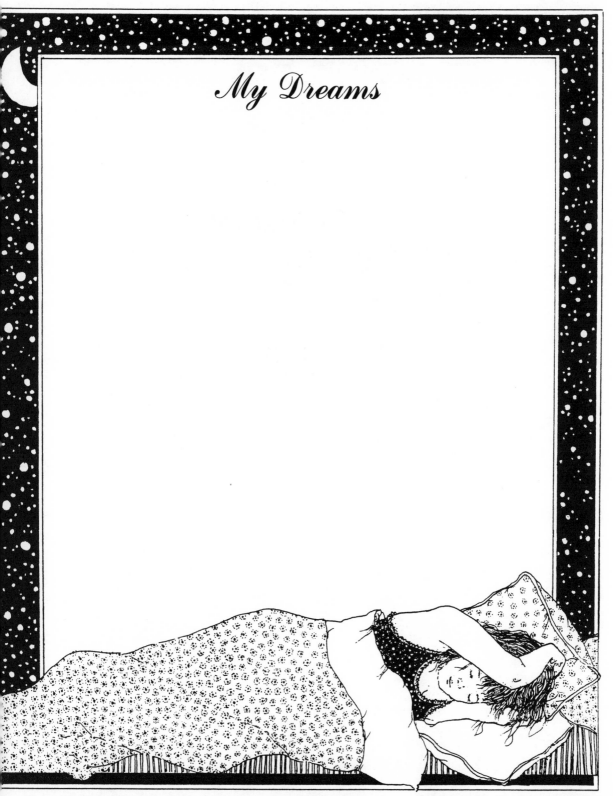

Your Growing Baby

The baby's muscles are getting stronger every week; if you haven't felt them before, you can certainly now feel his active movements. His legs are now in proportion with the rest of his body, and his movements are becoming increasingly sophisticated. The baby's kicking, punching, and tumbling will be a pretty constant part of your life for the next twenty weeks of pregnancy!

Your baby is growing rapidly and has reached about ten inches in length, which is half of what he'll probably measure at birth. This rapid growth will soon slow down. By the end of this month, the baby weighs about twelve ounces.

My Thoughts

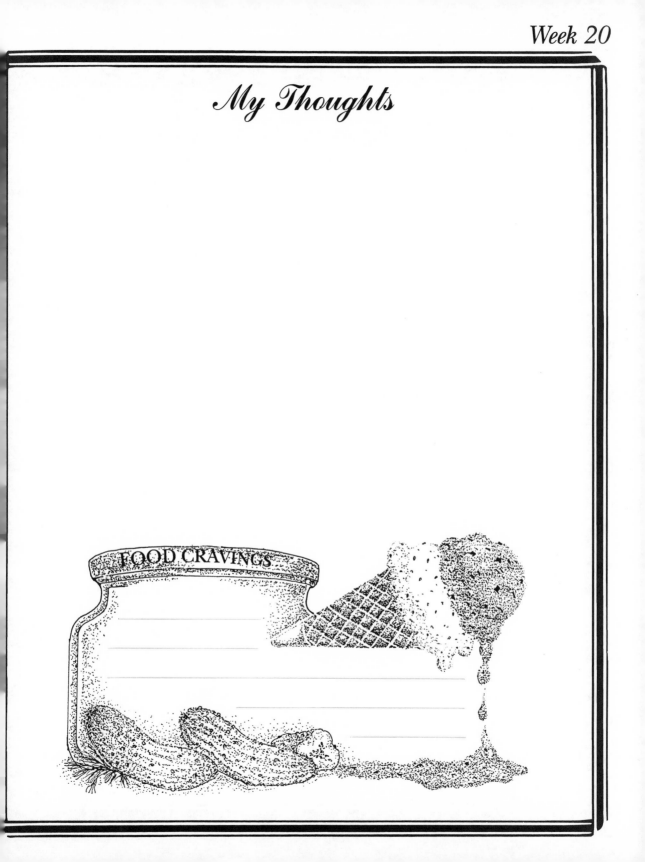

FOOD CRAVINGS

If I've had a baby before, what seems different this time?

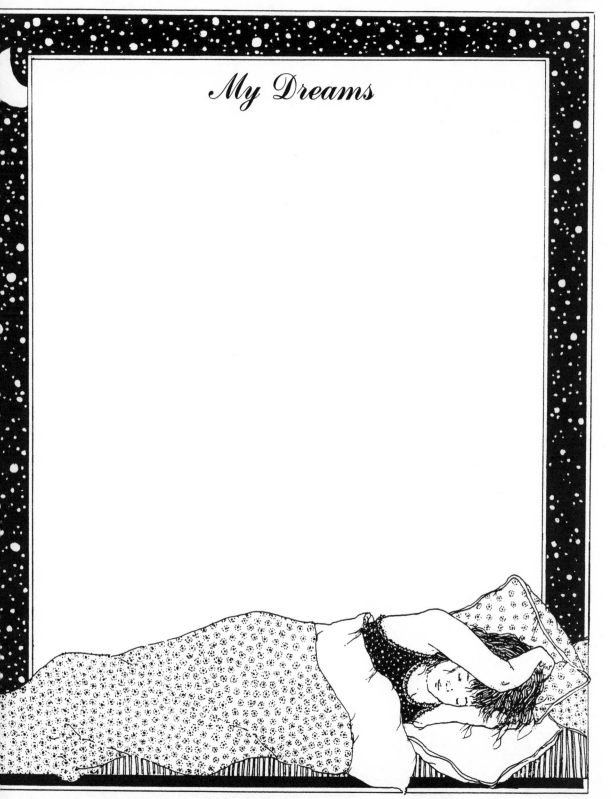

My Dreams

My Fifth-Month (20 Week) Doctor Visit

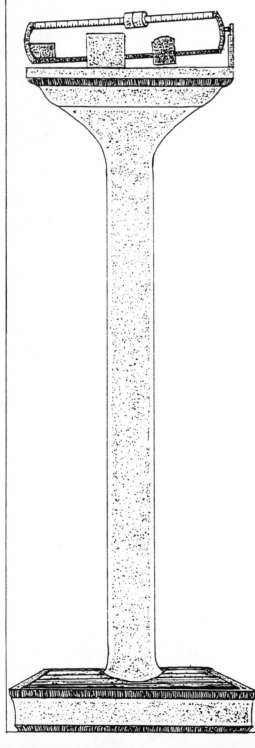

Weight _____ lbs.

Pounds gained since last visit _____ lbs.

Fundal height _____

Blood pressure _____

Urine (sugar, protein?) _____

Other tests? _____

Thigh measurement: *My (left/right) thigh is* _____

inches (_____ *inches more than last month).*

My Disappearing Waist

My waist is now _____ *inches*

(_____ *inches more than last month).*

Comments or Instructions from My Care Giver(s):

_____

_____

_____

_____

Questions I Want to Remember to Ask:

_____

_____

_____

_____

Reminder: Ask my practitioner whether I need to see my dentist around this point in my pregnancy, since a woman gums are more prone to infection when she is expecting.

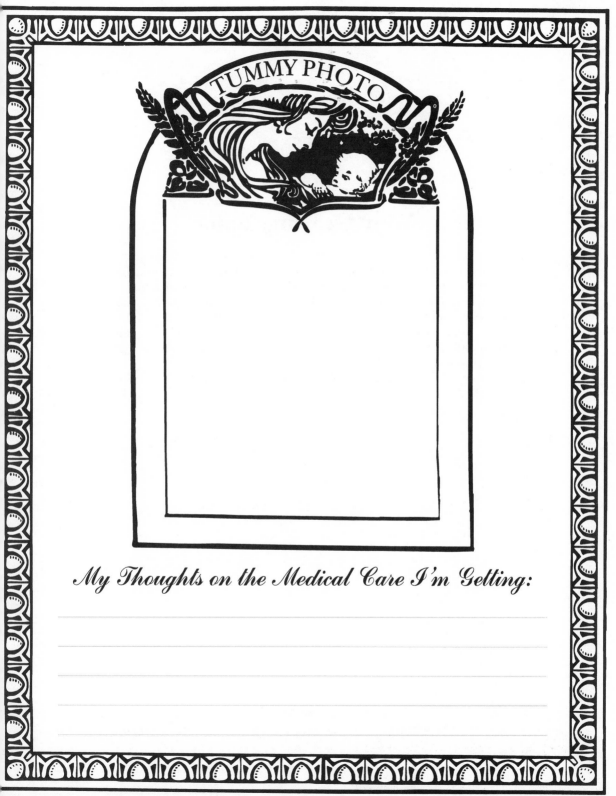

TUMMY PHOTO

My Thoughts on the Medical Care I'm Getting:

Your Growing Baby

In the past few weeks, *vernix* (a white, greasy substance) has been forming on your baby's delicate, newly formed skin to protect her from the liquid environment she has to live in all these months. From this point in your pregnancy, the vernix serves to protect the baby's skin from the increasing concentration of her urine in the amniotic fluid. By the time your baby is ready to be born, most of the vernix will have dissolved. However, some vernix will still be there to lubricate your baby's journey down the birth canal during labor and delivery.

Your baby has now reached about eleven inches and weighs just under a pound.

Getting to Know My Baby

Have I noticed when the baby is most active? Are there things I do that make her more or less likely to move around or kick?

If I have a job, what decisions have I made about altering my work once I'm a mother? What has my employer's reaction been?

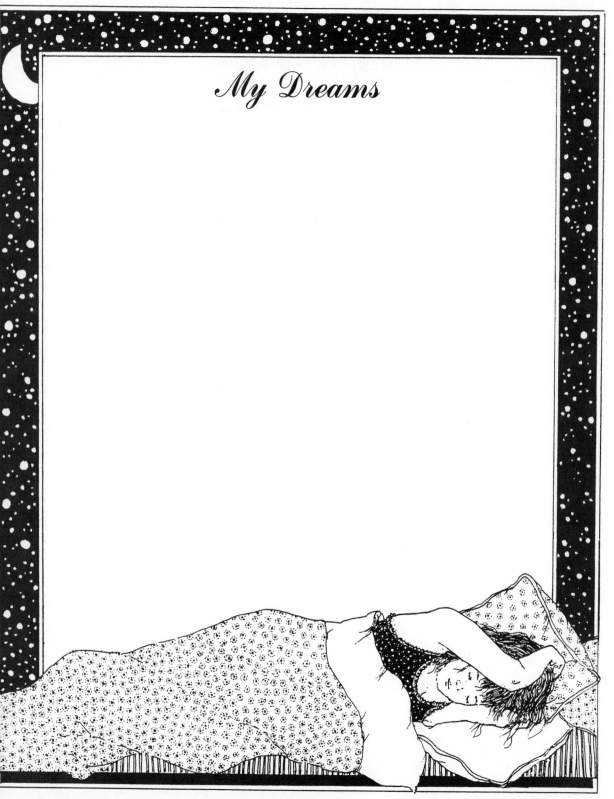

My Dreams

Your Growing Baby

The baby's body has started to produce white blood cells. These are essential in order for the baby to be able to combat disease and infection.

If your baby is a girl, her internal organs of reproduction, the vagina and uterus, have formed by now.

The baby is moving vigorously, and you may notice that she responds to your touch or sounds that reach her. A loud noise can make her jump or kick. If you haven't been aware of it before, you may feel a jerking motion inside you, which is the baby having hiccups.

And by this week your baby's tongue is fully developed.

Your baby has grown to about twelve inches long and weighs about one pound.

My Thoughts

OLD WIVES' TALES AND ADVICE

If a baby is carried high, she'll be a girl;
if you are carrying low, you will have a boy.

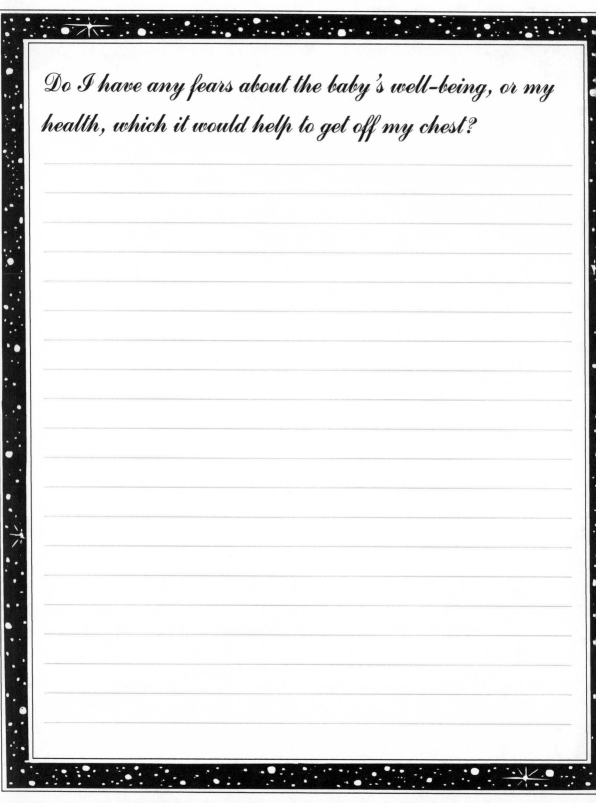

Do I have any fears about the baby's well-being, or my health, which it would help to get off my chest?

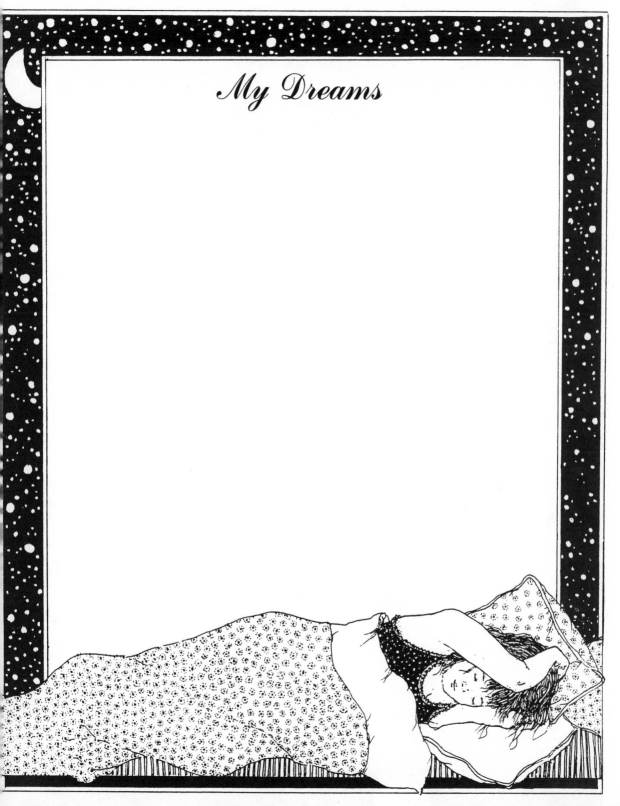

My Dreams

Your Growing Baby

Up until this point in your pregnancy, the baby's skin has been transparent, with the blood vessels visible through it; now it becomes opaque. His skin is extremely wrinkled, with loose folds, almost as though he hasn't grown into it, because there aren't yet any fat deposits underneath his skin. Creases have begun to appear on his fingertips and the palms of his hands. By next week his fingerprints and toeprints will be visible.

You can hear the baby's heartbeat through a stethoscope, and your husband may even be able to hear the baby's heart by putting his ear directly against your stomach.

My Thoughts

Names and Nicknames

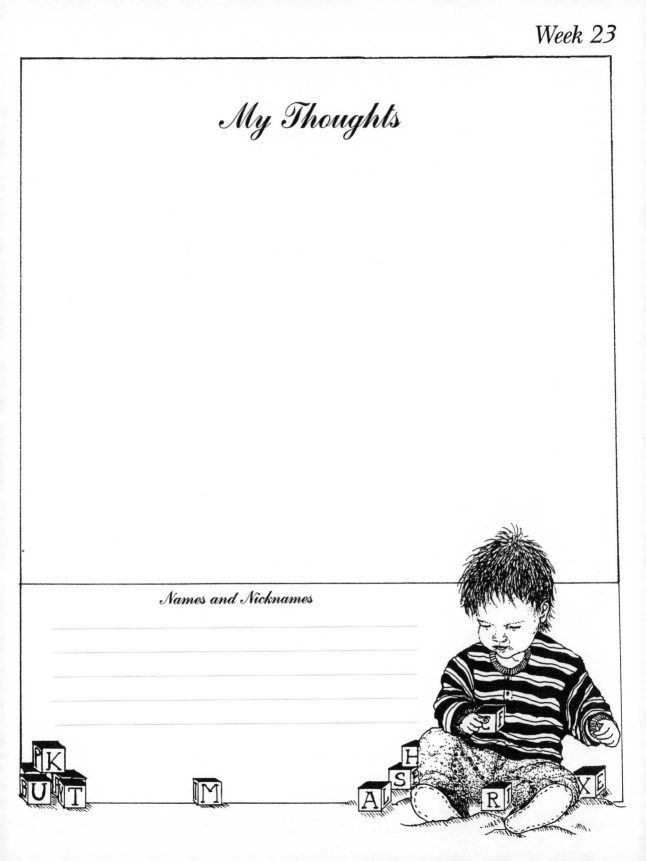

In what ways do I think parenthood is going to alter my partner? Has he talked about making changes in his lifestyle, like giving up dangerous or expensive hobbies? Has my husband talked about getting more involved in home care and baby care?

My Dreams

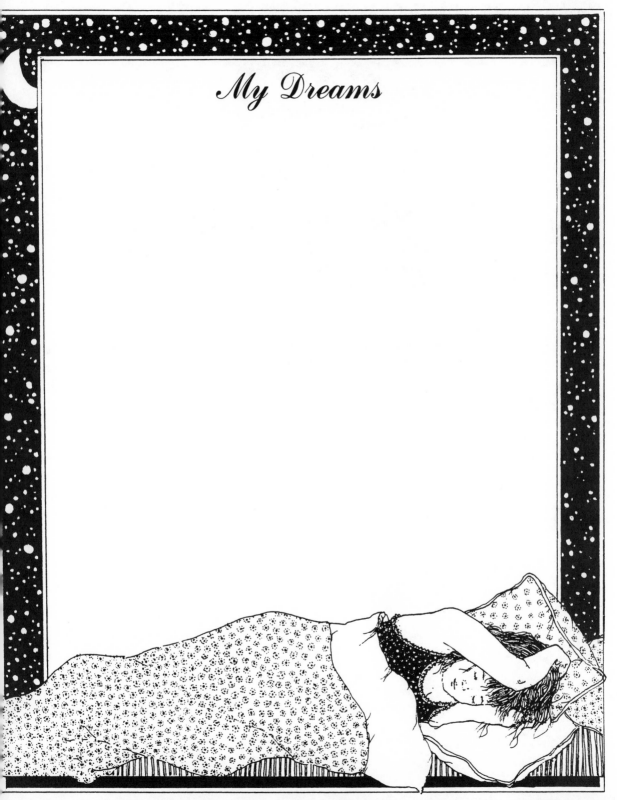

Your Growing Baby

By this week the baby's hearing system is perfectly developed; the organs of balance located in the inner ear have developed to the full dimension they'll have for life. Because water is a better sound conductor than air, the baby in utero can hear, although with distortions. Your baby reacts to sound; her pulse rate increases, and she'll move in rhythm to music she hears.

By the end of the baby's sixth month in your uterus, she is thirteen inches long and weighs about one pound two ounces.

My Thoughts

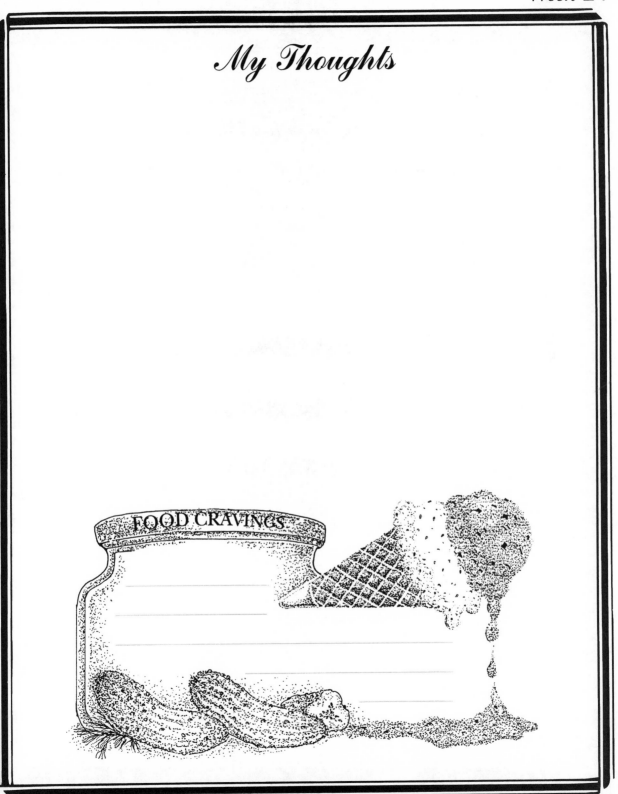

FOOD CRAVINGS

Has being pregnant changed my perception of myself, as either a woman, a wife, a daughter, or a part of the work force? How do I feel about those changes?

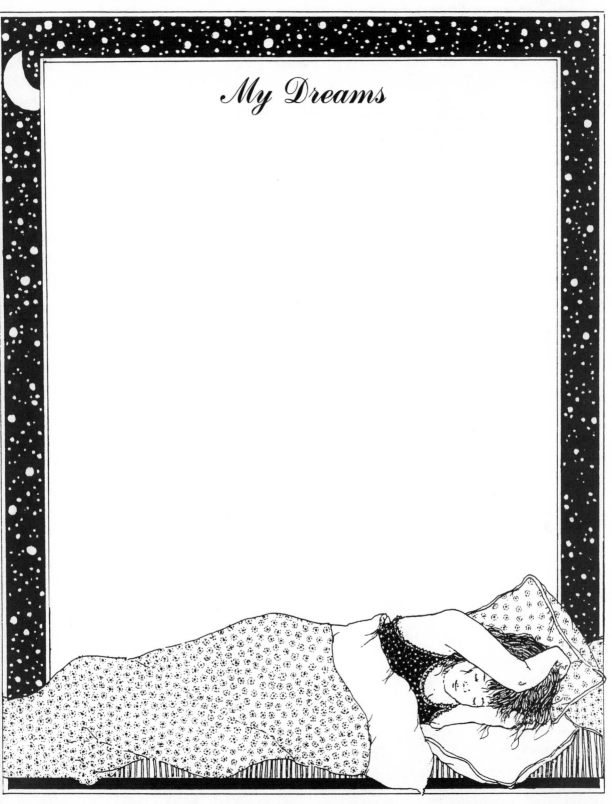

My Dreams

My Sixth-Month (24 Week) Doctor Visit

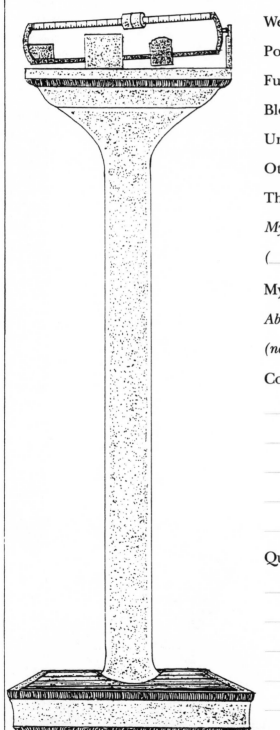

Weight _____ lbs.

Pounds gained since last visit _____ lbs.

Fundal height _____

Blood pressure _____

Urine (sugar, protein?) _____

Other tests? _____

Thigh measurement:

My (left/right) thigh is _____ *inches*

*(*_____ *inches more than last month).*

My Disappearing Waist

About that waist I used to have . . . .

(now it's _____ *inches bigger than last month).*

Comments or Instructions from My Care Giver(s):

_____

_____

_____

_____

_____

Questions I Want to Remember to Ask:

_____

_____

_____

_____

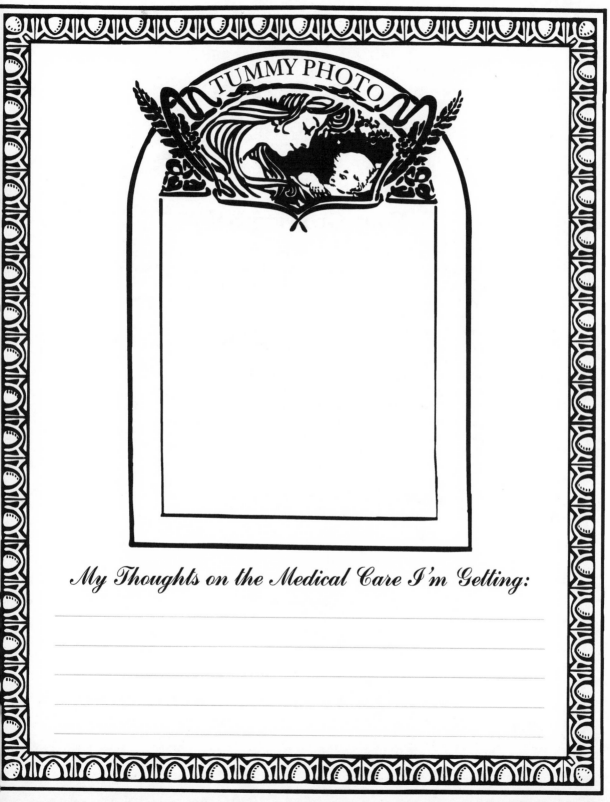

TUMMY PHOTO

My Thoughts on the Medical Care I'm Getting:

Your Growing Baby

The baby's hands are active now, and his muscular coordination has developed so that he's able to get his thumb into his mouth. Thumb sucking calms the baby and strengthens jaw and cheek muscles.

Although he's probably been hiccuping for some time, by this week he has a new skill: now he can cry!

Your baby's bone centers are beginning to harden.

At this point in your pregnancy, his growth is slow and steady. The baby's body is fattening up and growing at a faster pace than his head, which until now has been disproportionately large. The baby's body is getting long and thin, with fat deposits now building up under the skin.

In the last week your baby has grown about half an inch and added some weight. He now measures fourteen inches and weighs around one pound four ounces.

Getting to Know My Baby

What clues has my baby given me about her temperament?

How have I handled the emotional highs and lows of pregnancy? And how has my mate dealt with my emotions?

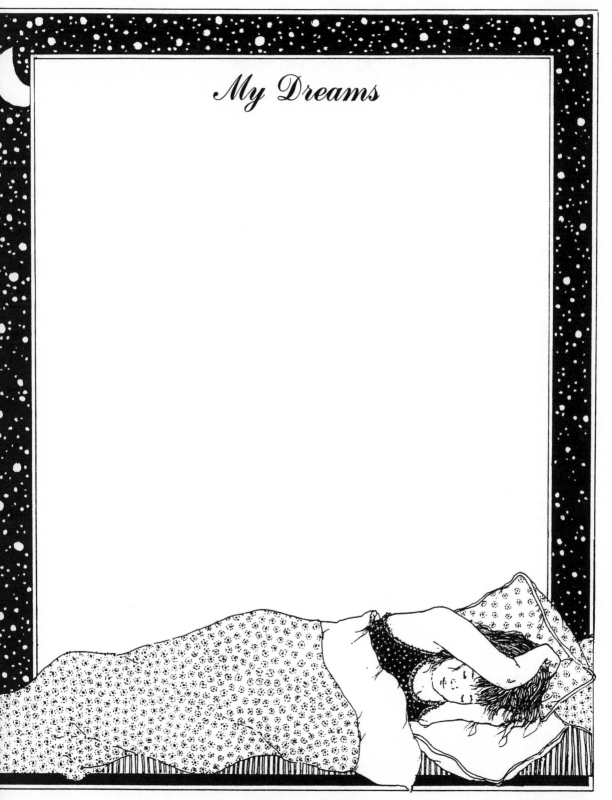

My Dreams

Your Growing Baby

Recordings of the baby's brain waves at the beginning of the last trimester (the sixth month of your pregnancy) show that the baby has rapid eye movement (REM) sleep, which in adults is associated with dreaming. This means that your unborn baby may be dreaming now.

The branches of your baby's lungs (the bronchi) are developing, although his lungs won't be fully formed until after he's born. However, if your baby were born prematurely at this point, there's a good chance his lungs would be able to function.

The placenta's usefulness begins to diminish during this month, and the amount of amniotic fluid decreases as the baby gets bigger.

My Thoughts

OLD WIVES' TALES AND ADVICE

Eat spicy food and your baby will grow hair.

Whether I know the sex of my baby or not, what do I think are some of the pluses and minuses of having either a boy or a girl?

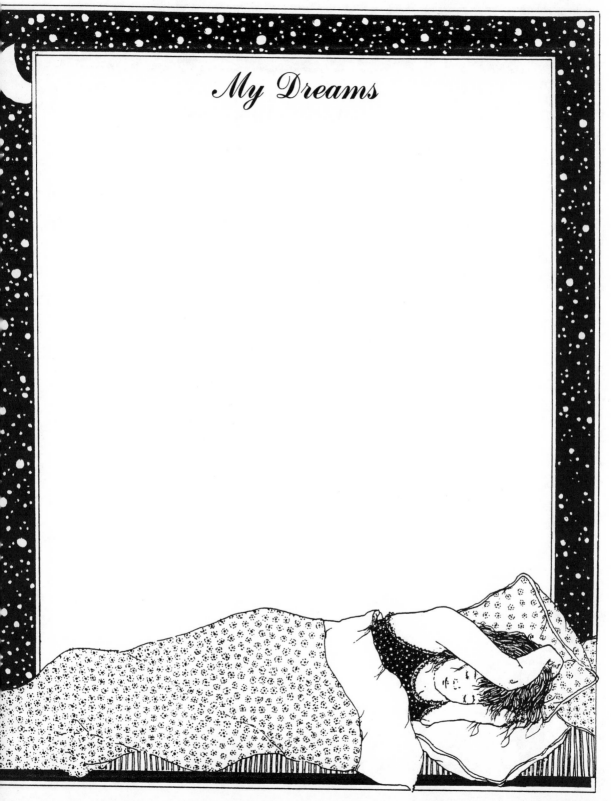

My Dreams

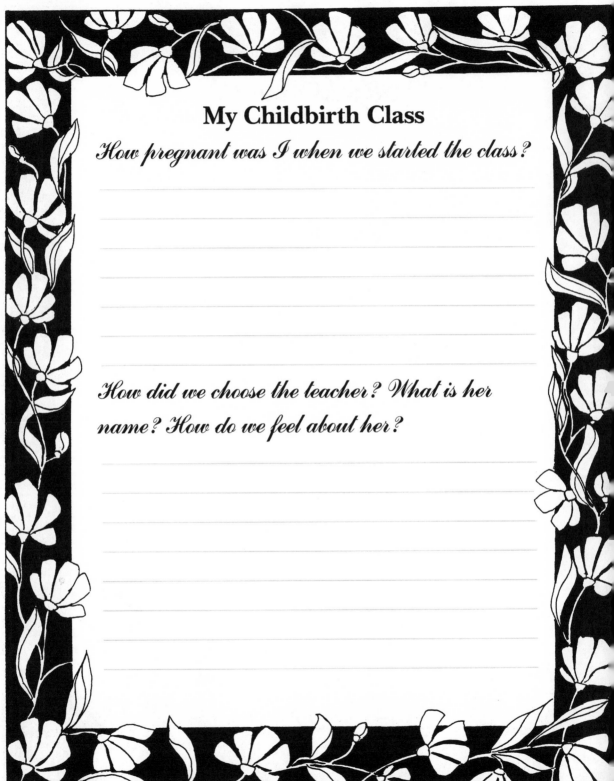

My Childbirth Class

How pregnant was I when we started the class?

How did we choose the teacher? What is her name? How do we feel about her?

Going in, what presumptions do I have about childbirth techniques?

_____

_____

_____

What do I expect childbirth training to give me personally?

_____

_____

_____

_____

What part of the training do I believe will really make a difference in my childbirth experience?

_____

_____

_____

_____

Is there some aspect of childbirth training that I view as somewhat hocus-pocus?

Was my husband enthusiastic or ambivalent about going to the class?

Have we practiced together regularly, or does one of us have to remind or nag the other?

_____

_____

_____

_____

Is there anybody in the class I feel I can relate to and might want to strike up a friendship with?

_____

_____

_____

Have I considered asking the teacher if she would be willing to assist at my birth?

_____

_____

_____

Your Growing Baby

The membranes that covered your baby's eyes separate this week, and her eyelids begin to part. She can open her eyes and look around for the first time. It isn't always dark inside your uterus, since bright sunlight or artificial light can filter through the uterine wall. At this stage of development, a baby's eyes are almost blue: her true eye coloring will generally not fully develop until a few months after birth. (A few babies' eyes do turn brown soon after birth.)

She now also has fully developed delicate eyebrows and eyelashes.

Your baby now weighs about two pounds, although her length has not changed much in the last two weeks: she's still about fourteen inches long.

My Thoughts

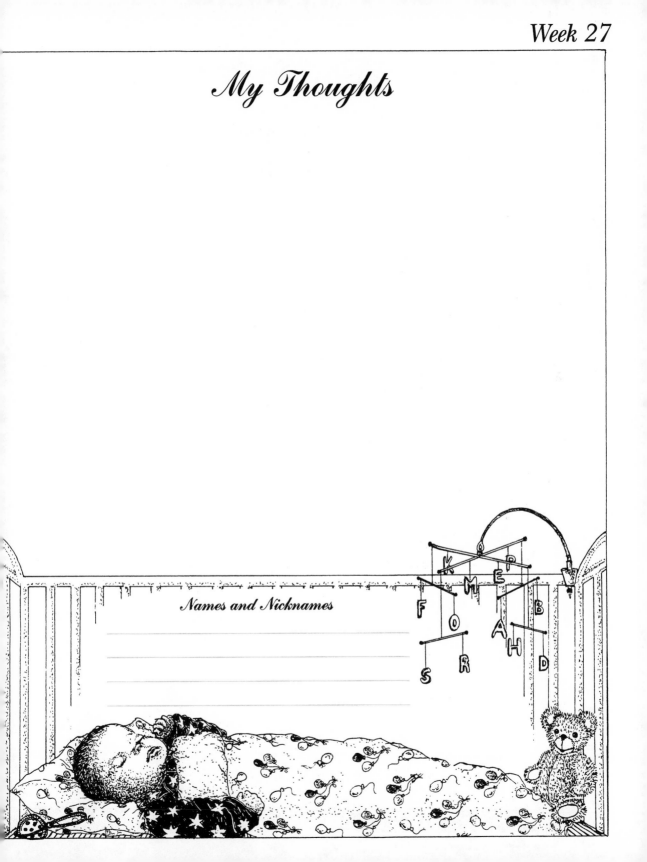

Names and Nicknames

What kinds of daydreams and fantasies have I been having about my child and the life we're going to share?

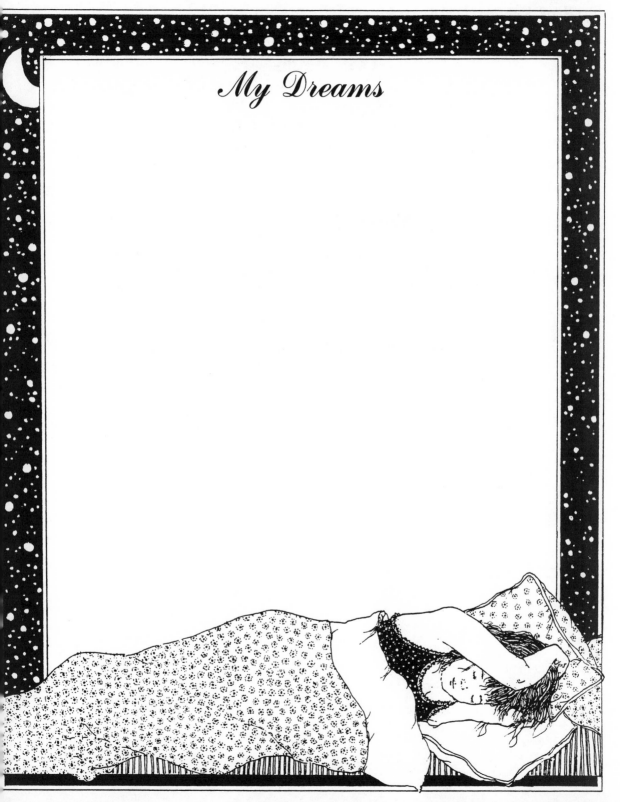

My Dreams

Your Growing Baby

If your baby were to be born prematurely now, he's matured sufficiently to be able to live independently. His lungs, the essential part of living outside the womb, are reaching maturity, although he might need medical help to breathe and maintain his body temperature.

By this twenty-eighth week of pregnancy, a boy's testicles have descended into his scrotum.

The baby has put on more than a pound in this seventh month, for a total weight of about two pounds four ounces. His length has reached fifteen inches.

My Thoughts

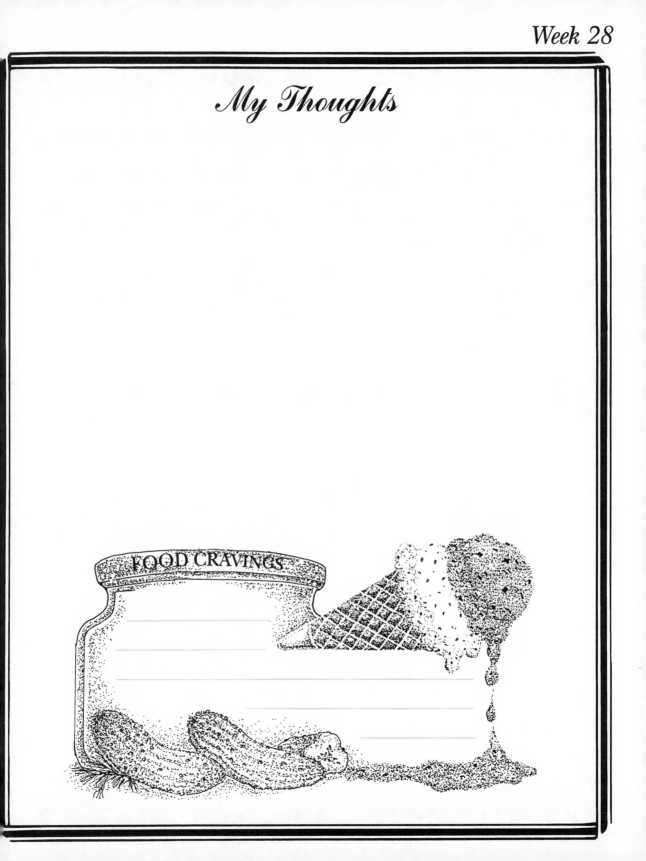

FOOD CRAVINGS

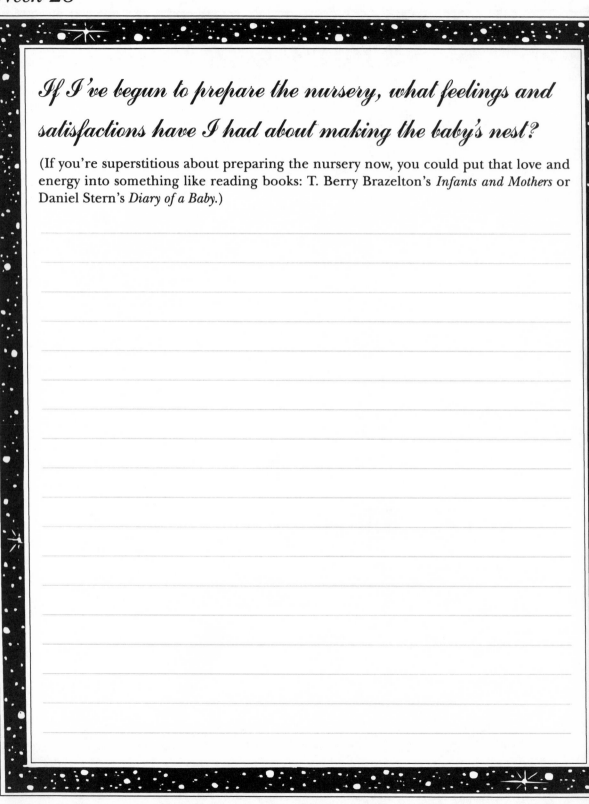

If I've begun to prepare the nursery, what feelings and satisfactions have I had about making the baby's nest?

(If you're superstitious about preparing the nursery now, you could put that love and energy into something like reading books: T. Berry Brazelton's *Infants and Mothers* or Daniel Stern's *Diary of a Baby*.)

My Dreams

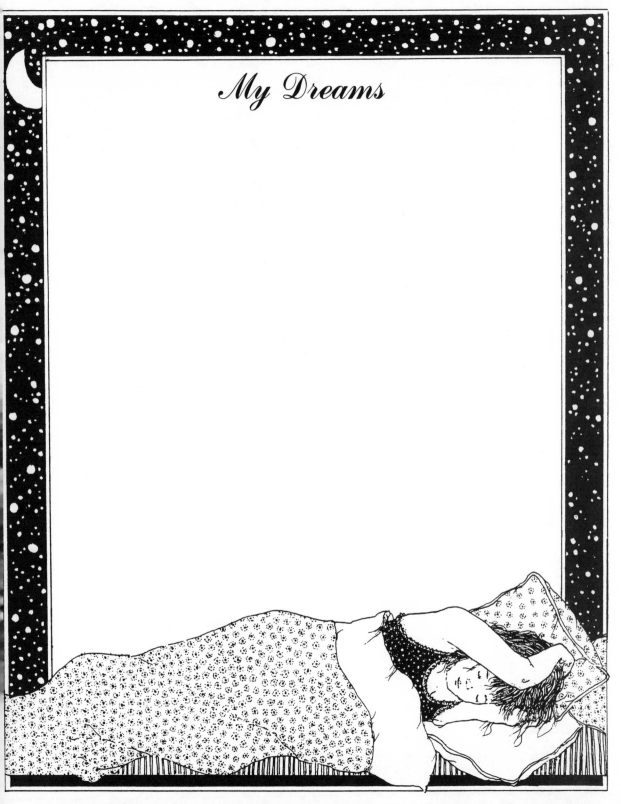

My Seventh-Month (28 Week) Doctor Visit

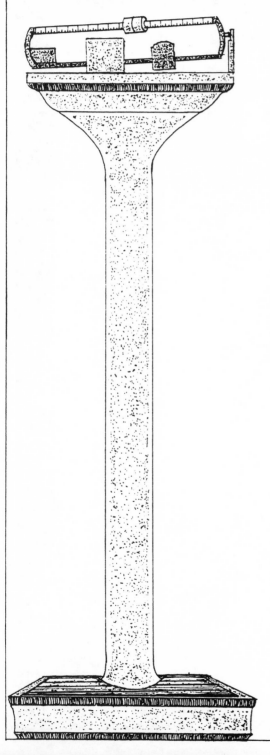

Weight _____ lbs.

Pounds gained since last visit _____ lbs.

Fundal height _____

Blood pressure _____

Urine (sugar, protein?) _____

Other tests? _____

Thigh measurement:

My (left/right) thigh is _____ inches

(_____ inches more than last month).

My Disappearing Waist

Okay, so it's not a waist anymore! Still, let's measure how

many inches it is _____, and how many inches bigger

than it was last month _____.

Comments or Instructions from My Care Giver(s):

_____

_____

_____

Questions I Want to Remember to Ask:

_____

_____

_____

_____

TUMMY PHOTO

My Thoughts on the Medical Care I'm Getting:

Your Growing Baby

The baby can hear even more by this stage in your pregnancy; previously he could mainly hear vibrations, but now the nerve endings in his ears that enable him to hear sounds are connected. Although there are indications that some babies' hearing starts to develop earlier, by now most babies can definitely hear distinct sounds. Your baby can hear your voice now, which researchers know because his heart rate increases when his mother or father speaks. This means your baby may even be able to recognize your voice after birth. Also, your baby can hear music now, although it has to be played quite loudly since his ears are plugged by water and vernix. After he's born, when the baby hears music you played before birth, he may show he recognizes it by becoming less active while he listens.

Your baby is gaining about seven ounces a week and now weighs about two pounds eleven ounces. His weekly growth in length is a bit under half an inch, so by this week he measures just a little more than fifteen inches.

Getting to Know My Baby

Is there a time of day when my baby is most active or responsive?

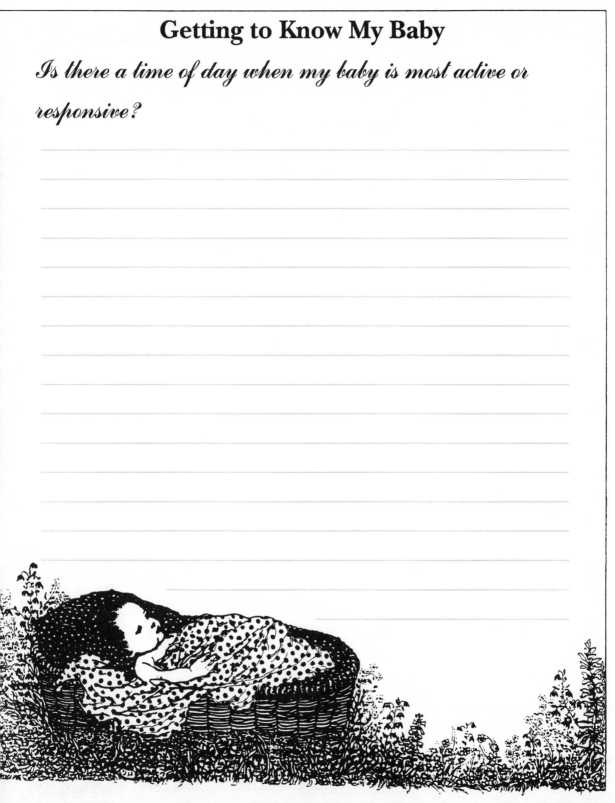

Has food generally been a problem for me during pregnancy? Do I want a lot of it and worry about gaining weight, or am I turned off by food and worry about nourishing the baby?

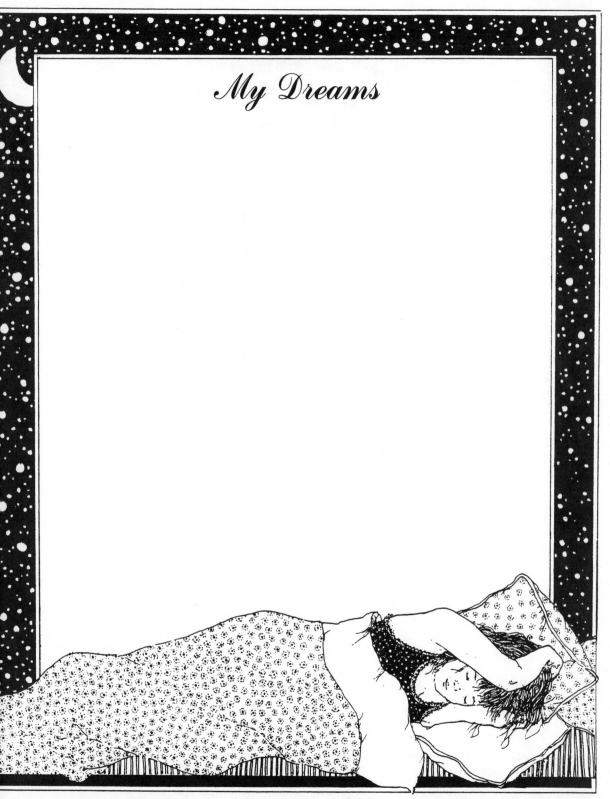

My Dreams

Your Growing Baby

Your baby now fills almost all the space in your uterus. She may be lying with her head up or she may still have room to do somersaults. However, at any time from now on, your baby will probably turn upside down into a vertex (head down) position. You'll probably feel more comfortable when her head is nestled in your bony pelvis.

Your baby's brain is growing rapidly, and she's practicing opening her eyes and breathing.

She weighs about three pounds two ounces this week.

My Thoughts

OLD WIVES' TALES AND ADVICE

*A pregnant woman should never try to make preserves,
because they will spoil.*

Have I been having conflicting feelings about pregnancy and motherhood? Do ambivalent feelings make me feel frightened or guilty instead of being able to accept them as normal?

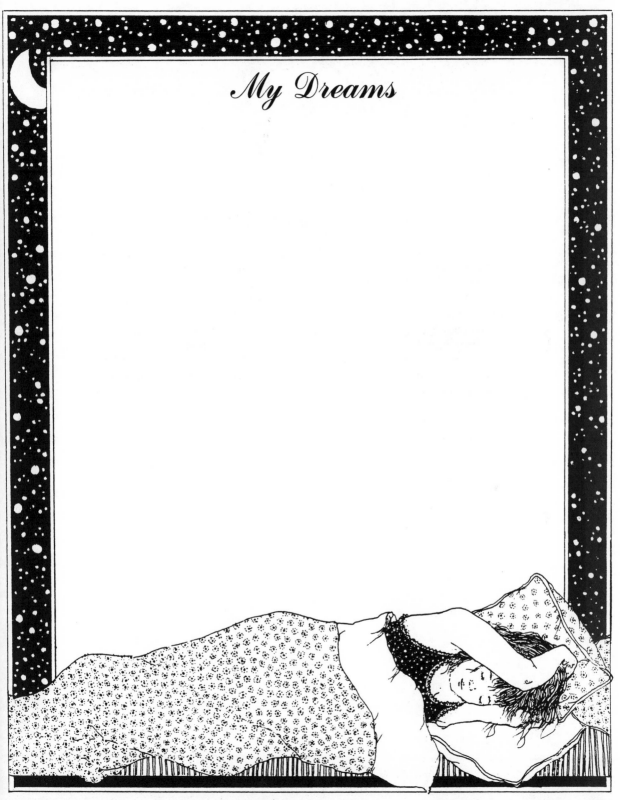

My Dreams

Your Growing Baby

Your baby begins to move less inside you as she runs out of room. She's probably lying in a curled-up position, with her knees bent, her chin resting on her chest, and her arms and legs crossed.

If she hasn't turned upside down into a head-down position by this week, she will be likely to do so in the next seven days; most babies turn into a vertex position to be born head-first. If she doesn't turn, your doctor or midwife may try to turn the baby around by manipulating her from the outside.

During this week the air sacs inside the baby's lungs become lined with a layer of cells that produce a liquid called *surfactant*. This material prevents the air sacs from collapsing when your baby first begins to breathe after birth.

This week your baby measures under sixteen inches and weighs about three pounds nine ounces.

My Thoughts

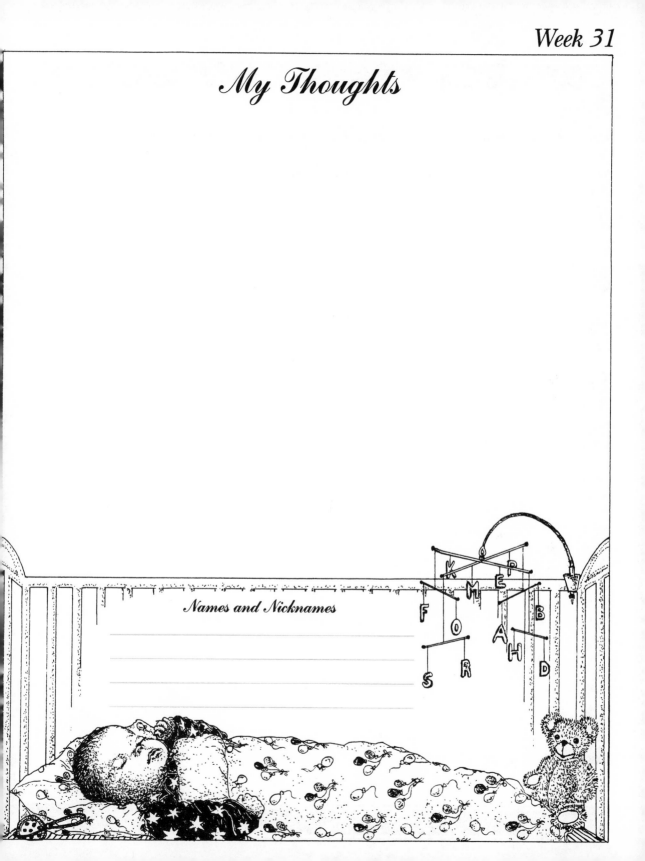

Names and Nicknames

What has being pregnant made me realize about the control that we sometimes like to think we have over our lives?

My Dreams

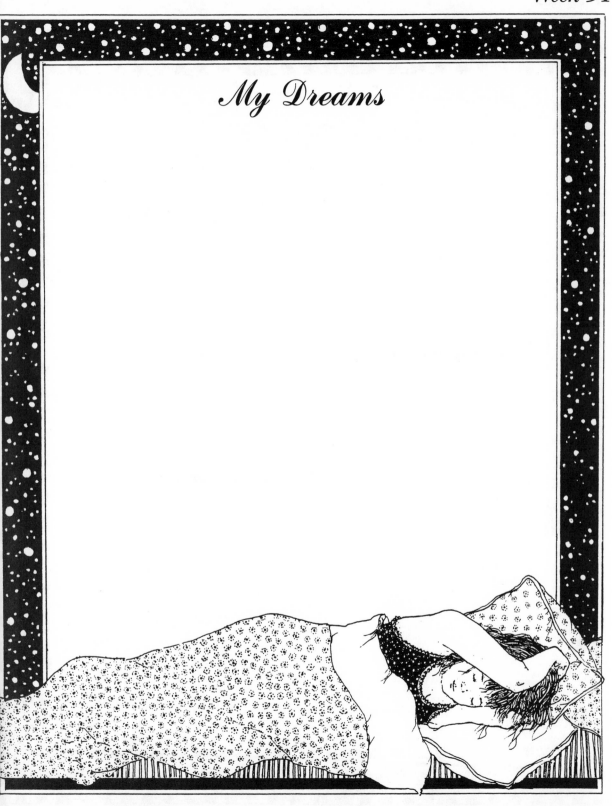

My Baby Shower

Where and when was the party?

Who was the hostess?

What was served?

Anything particular I'd like to record about the festivities?

Who Came, and What Gifts Did They Give the Baby?

(You can use this list to check off when you've written a thank-you note)

NAME	GIFT	THANKS

Your Growing Baby

The baby is now likely to have settled into a vertex position, where he will stay until birth. Smaller babies with more room to move can bounce between vertex and breech (bottom-down) positions for several more weeks. You will know if your baby has turned into the head-down position because instead of the baby's head pressing against your ribs, you'll feel his feet kicking against your rib cage. The baby's elbows and knees may be more visible as they press against the uterine wall.

Growth, especially of the brain, is great at this time.

As your baby grows plumper, the wrinkles in his skin fill out and he appears smoother. Both the lanugo and vernix that cover his skin begin to disappear around this time.

By the end of the eighth month the baby weighs about four pounds, although he probably doesn't grow significantly in length this week.

My Thoughts

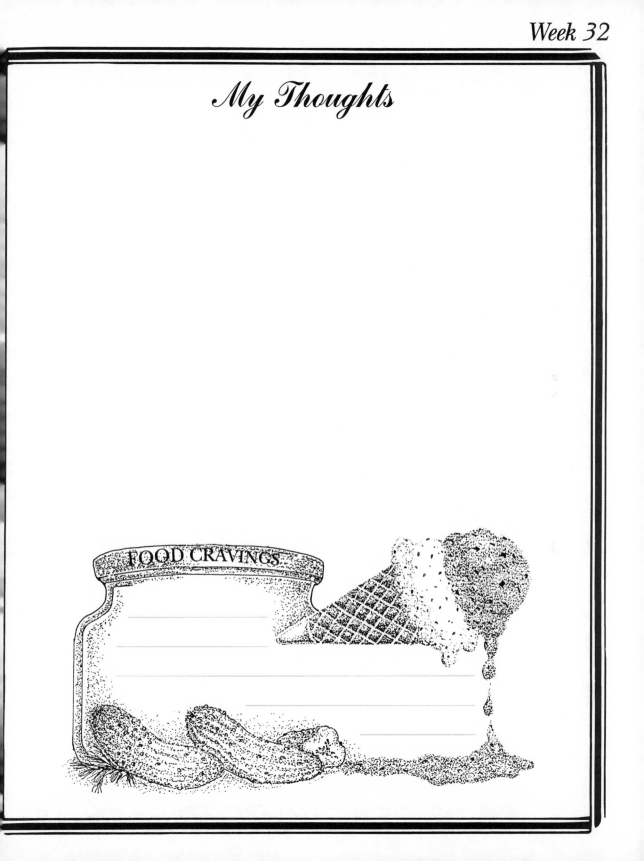

FOOD CRAVINGS

Now that I'm getting close to being a mother, what thoughts have I been having about my childhood?

My Dreams

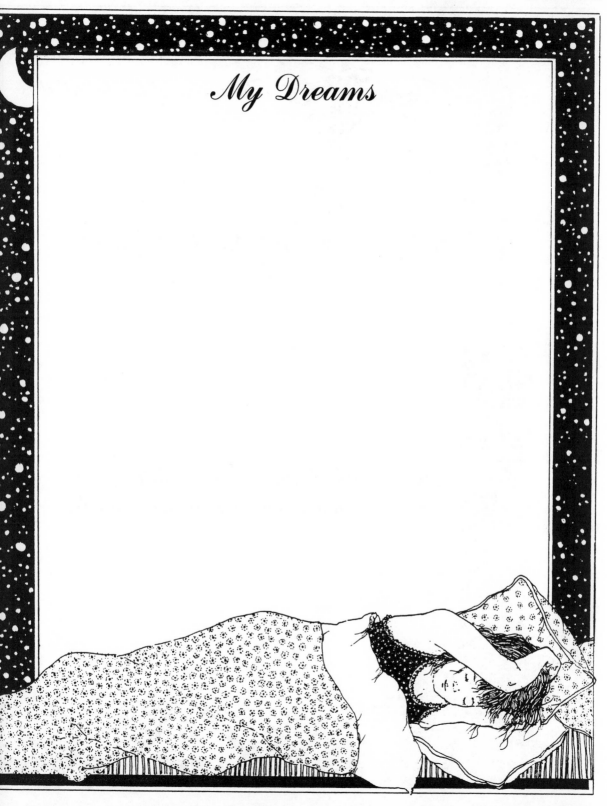

My Tour of the Hospital

The name of the hospital is

_____

_____

_____

_____

What have I heard about the hospital?

_____

_____

_____

_____

_____

_____

_____

Have I asked other women who've given birth there what their experiences were like?

_____

_____

_____

_____

What aspects of the labor and delivery area am I interested in finding out about?

What does a hospital represent to me personally?

Are there negative connotations to being in a hospital for me that I should be aware of and work out ahead of time so that they don't interfere with my ability to have a positive experience?

Does a hospital represent anything negative to my husband or remind him of any previous medical experiences that might get in his way of having a good birth experience?

What questions do I want to be sure to ask on the hospital tour?

My Eighth-Month (32 Week) Doctor Visit

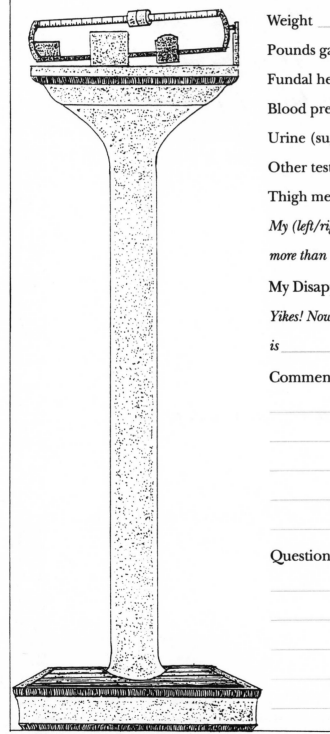

Weight _____ lbs.

Pounds gained since last visit _____ lbs.

Fundal height _____

Blood pressure _____

Urine (sugar, protein?) _____

Other tests? _____

Thigh measurement:

My (left/right) thigh is _____ inches (_____ inches more than last month).

My Disappearing Waist

Yikes! Now my waist has exploded to _____ inches, which is _____ inches more than just one month ago!

Comments or Instructions from My Care Giver(s):

_____

_____

_____

_____

Questions I Want to Remember to Ask:

_____

_____

_____

_____

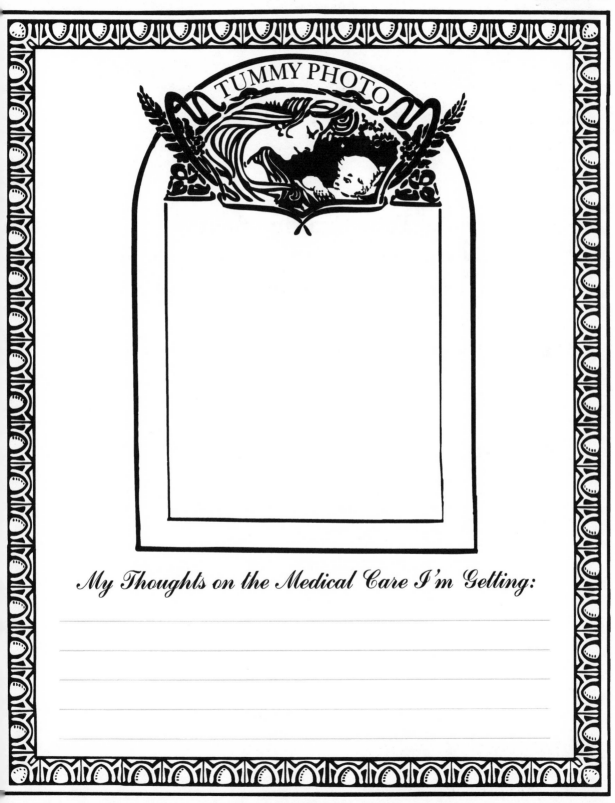

TUMMY PHOTO

My Thoughts on the Medical Care I'm Getting:

Your Growing Baby

Your baby's lungs are almost fully developed now, although she would probably be placed in an incubator if she were born now.

She's still on the thin side, but she's perfectly formed, with the proportions you'll see when she's born. She still doesn't have enough insulating fat deposits underneath her skin to keep warm outside your womb.

You may be more aware of her activities as she takes up more room inside you. Her movements can be vigorous at this point and may cause you discomfort, especially if her feet get caught under your ribs.

Your baby now weighs about four pounds seven ounces, and measures more than one foot four inches.

Getting to Know My Baby

Do I feel closer to my baby at this point, as though we are forming a bond?

Is there anything my husband does that gets a special reaction from our baby, like talking to her or massaging her through my belly?

My Dreams

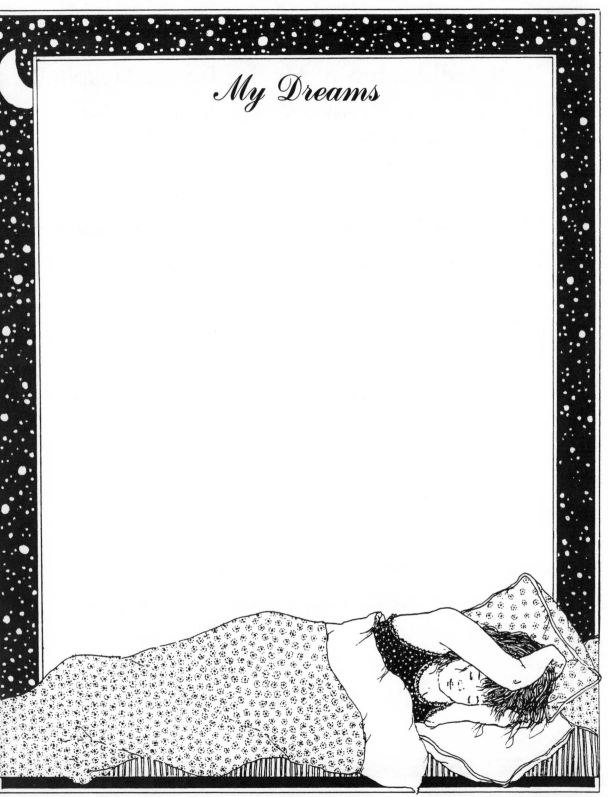

Revealed! Secrets of My Bag for the Hospital!

How many months before the due date did I start
preparing the bag? _____

_____

Where have I been keeping it? And have I changed where
I keep the bag as my due date gets nearer?

_____

_____

_____

What paraphernalia (like tennis balls, pillows) related to
childbirth classes is in the bag?

_____

_____

_____

What books or magazines did I pack—under the delusion
I'll have the time or energy to read in the hospital?!

_____

_____

_____

_____

What snacks and drinks am I putting in for my spouse?

*How many going-home outfits for the baby did I pack—
or how many times have I changed the ones I picked?!*

*Anything else I've got in the bag that I'd like
to reveal here?*

Your Growing Baby

Growth, especially of the brain, has been enormous in the past few weeks.

Most of the baby's systems are well developed, although her lungs may still be immature. She's probably trying to practice breathing using her lungs, but since no air is available, she swallows amniotic fluid into her windpipe, which can give her frequent hiccups.

The baby's eyes are usually slate color, and she is practicing blinking.

Her hair has been growing, and can be as much as two inches long by this week.

Your baby responds to familiar voices.

By this week, your baby weighs about four pounds fourteen ounces.

My Thoughts

OLD WIVES' TALES AND ADVICE

A baby born at the time of the new moon will be exceptionally strong and muscular.

Have we been practicing our childbirth techniques? If "yes," does the relaxation work? If "no," why not?

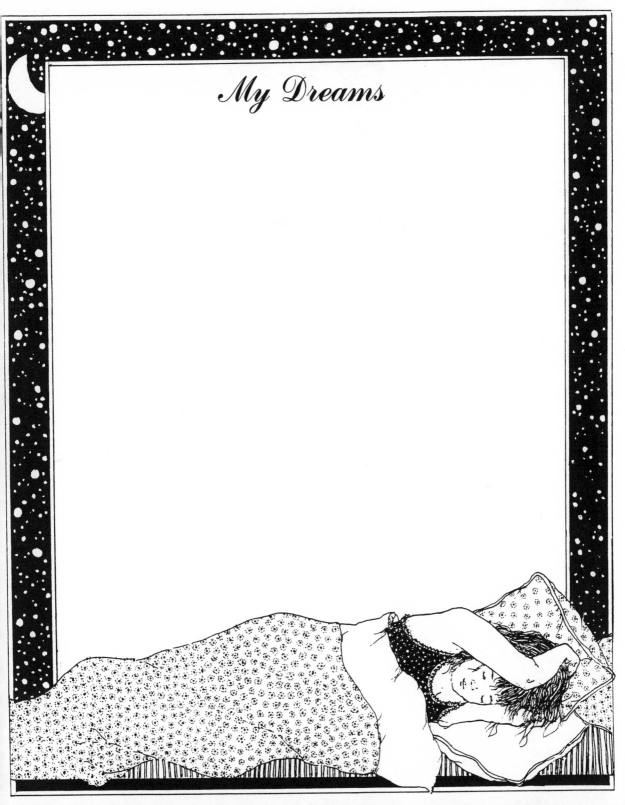

My Dreams

Your Growing Baby

Your baby is getting rounder day by day, losing his wrinkled appearance as he plumps up. Between this week and when he is born, he will continuously accumulate fat deposits beneath his skin. His skin is losing its redness and becoming pinker each day, too. Your baby weighs five pounds five ounces, and is just under one foot five inches.

My Thoughts

Names and Nicknames

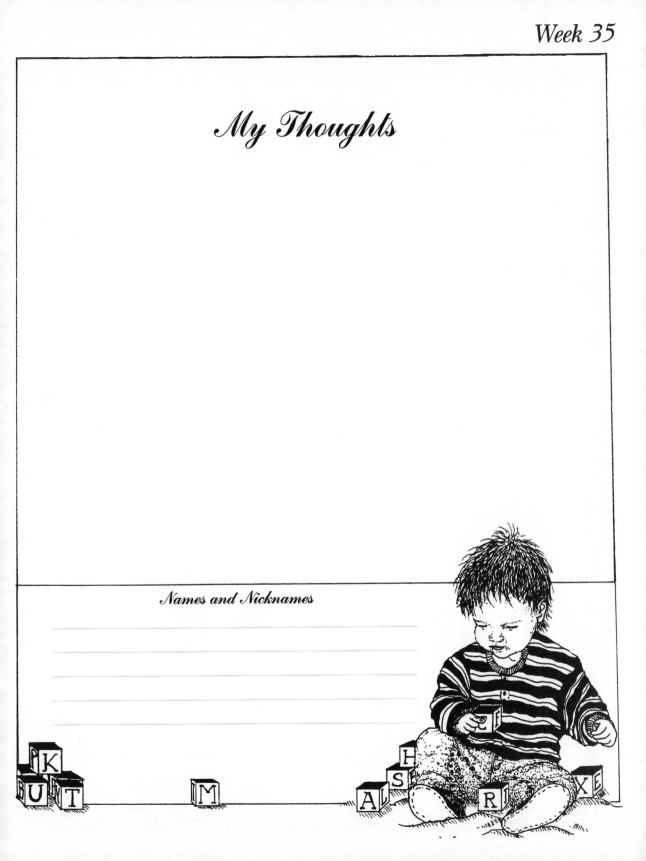

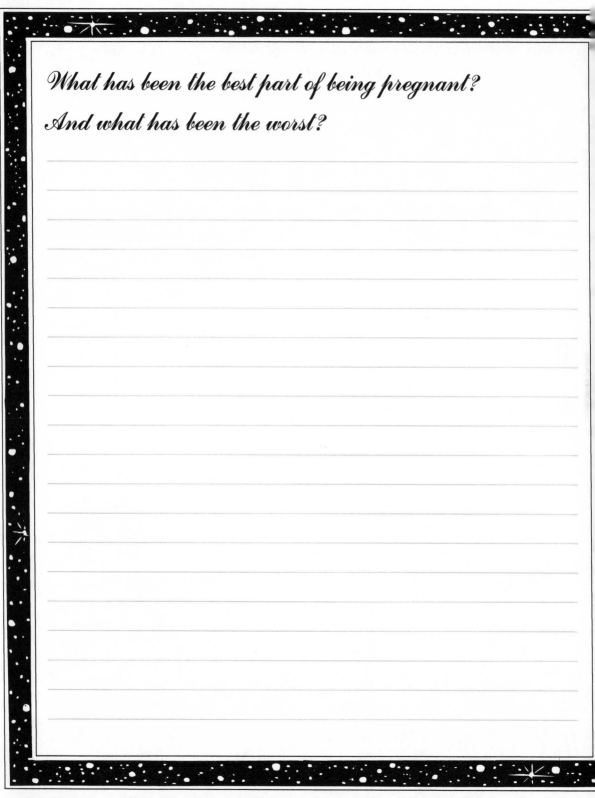

What has been the best part of being pregnant?
And what has been the worst?

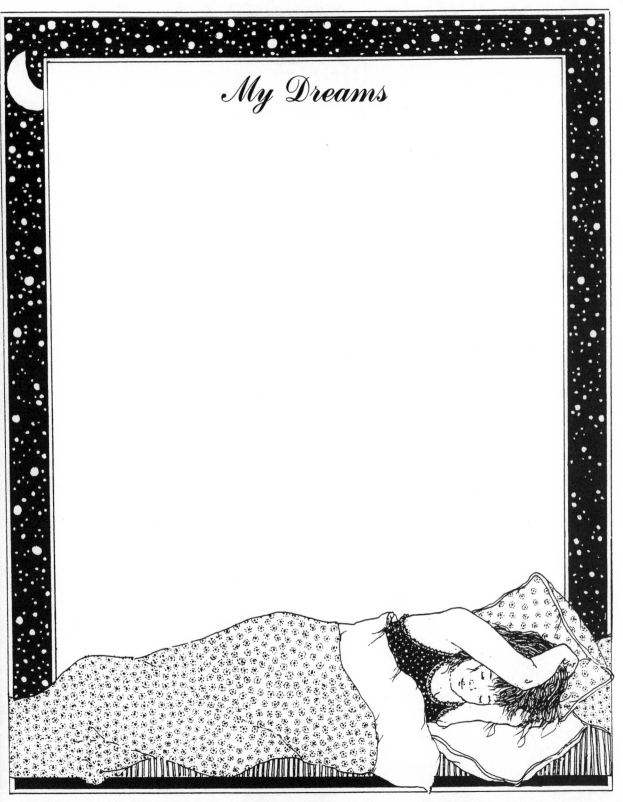

My Dreams

Week 36
(End of Ninth Month)

Your Growing Baby

By thirty-six weeks the baby is almost ready for birth; if he were born now, he would be premature but he would do well.

In this last trimester of your pregnancy, the baby has received antibodies from you and has gotten protection from whatever illnesses you've had, from measles to the common cold, or any diseases you've been immunized against, like polio or smallpox.

The baby's rate of growth is slowing down, although this is the time when he needs to get more plump to prepare himself for life on the outside. Fat cells are being deposited under the baby's skin every day.

During this month your baby has gained two pounds: he weighs five pounds twelve ounces, and his length is one foot six inches.

My Thoughts

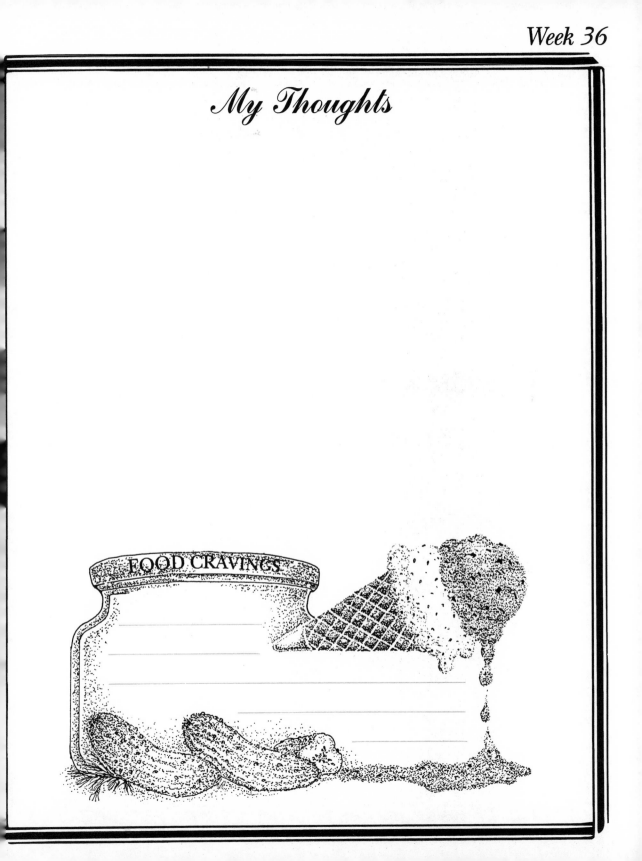

FOOD CRAVINGS

What fears do I have about how I am going to cope with labor and delivery?

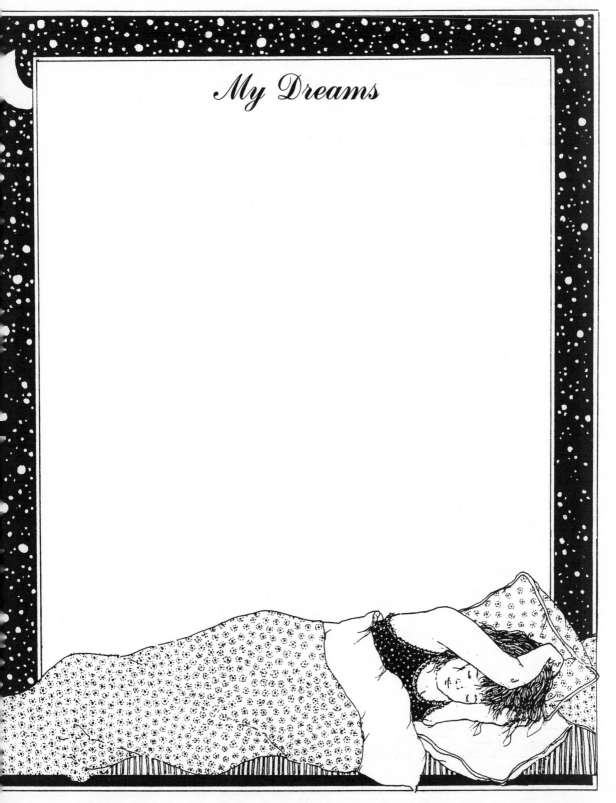

My Dreams

My Ninth-Month (36 Week) Doctor Visit

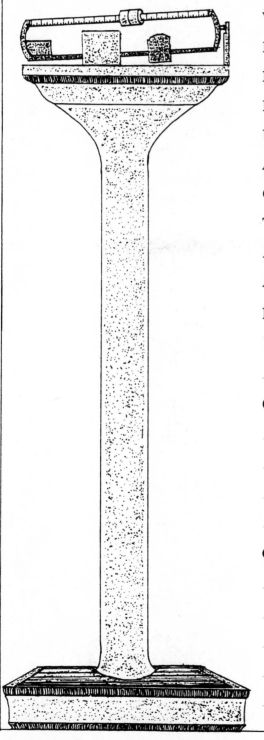

Weight _____ lbs.

Pounds gained since last visit _____ lbs.

Fundal height _____

Blood pressure _____

Urine (sugar, protein?) _____

Any effacement or dilation? _____

Other tests? _____

Thigh measurement:

My (left/right) thigh is _____ inches.

Any increase (_____ inches) from last month?

My Disappearing Waist

What waist?! Oh well, it's _____ inches, which is

_____ inches more than last month.

Comments or Instructions from My Care Giver(s):

_____

_____

_____

Questions I Want to Remember to Ask:

_____

_____

_____

_____

TUMMY PHOTO

My Thoughts on the Medical Care I'm Getting:

Your Growing Baby

The baby's toenails and fingernails have grown to the tips of her toes and fingers.

Her muscles have grown strong from vigorous motions of her arms and legs.

She continues to practice the movements of her lungs she'll need to breathe outside your body.

All your baby's organs are now almost fully mature: only her lungs need a little longer to complete their development.

If your baby is in a vertex position, her head has probably dropped into your pelvis by this week.

Getting to Know My Baby

What do I imagine the baby will like the most about me,
and what will he like the least?

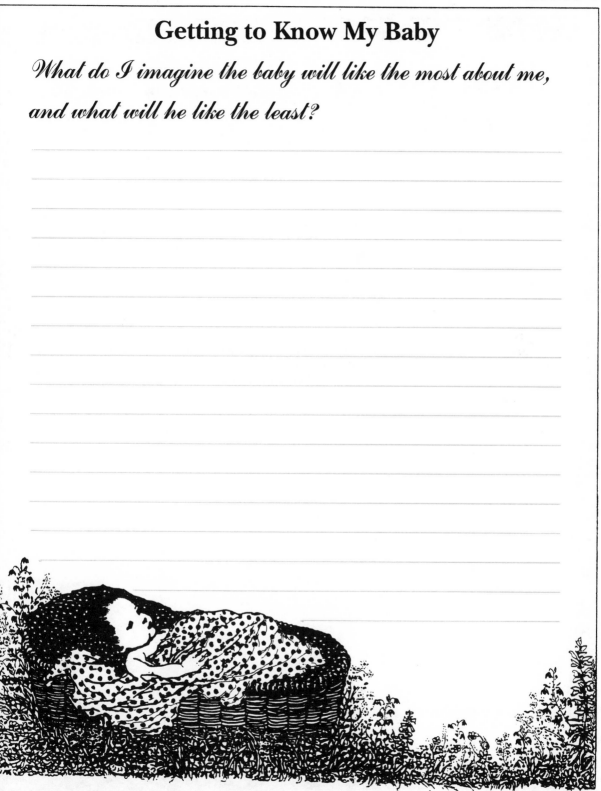

What thoughts have I been having about my own mother as I get closer to being a mother myself?

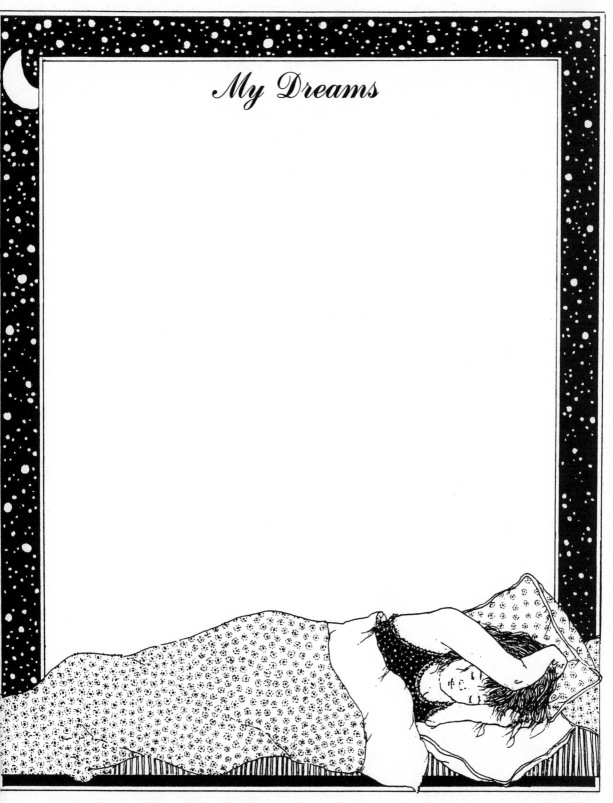

My Dreams

My (37 Week) Doctor Visit

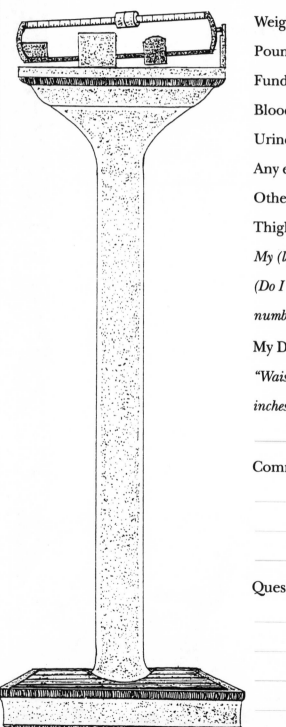

Weight _____ lbs.

Pounds gained since last visit _____ lbs.

Fundal height _____

Blood pressure _____

Urine (sugar, protein?) _____

Any effacement or dilation? _____

Other tests? _____

Thigh measurement:

My (left/right) thigh is now _____ inches.

(Do I really have the courage to keep doing this, hoping the

number won't get higher?!)

My Disappearing Waist

"Waist" is a strange word for it, but there are _____

inches now around that basketball I swallowed! And it's

_____ inches bigger than it was last month!

Comments or Instructions from My Care Giver(s):

_____

_____

_____

Questions I Want to Remember to Ask:

_____

_____

_____

_____

TUMMY PHOTO

My Thoughts on the Medical Care I'm Getting:

Your Growing Baby

The baby's reflexes have become coordinated so that he can blink and close his eyes, turn his head, grasp firmly, and respond to sounds, light, and touch. He can differentiate between light and dark and can see more if there is direct sunlight (or another source of bright light) shining directly on your stomach.

The fine lanugo hair covering his body has been falling out, and this process speeds up this week, although some may remain on his shoulders, in the folds of his skin, and maybe even on the back of his ears. Whatever lanugo is left when he's born will fall out in the early postpartum days.

My Thoughts

OLD WIVES' TALES AND ADVICE

During childbirth the mother's head should always be toward the north,
which brings luck to the baby.

*What pediatricians have my husband and I interviewed,
and how did we like them?*

My Dreams

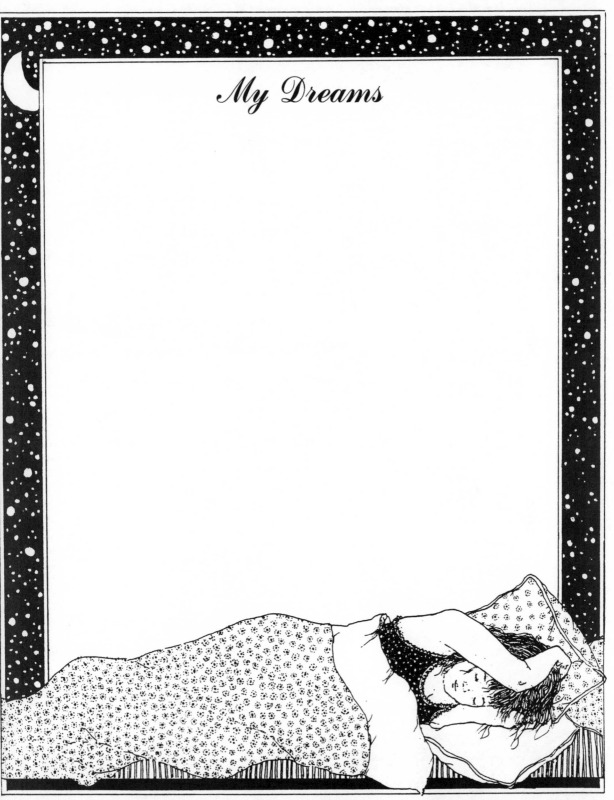

My (38 Week) Doctor Visit

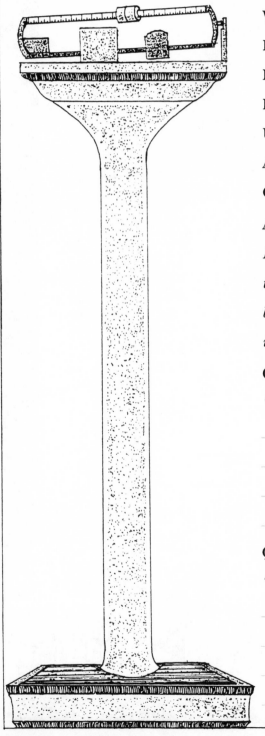

Weight _____ lbs.

Pounds gained since last visit _____ lbs.

Fundal height _____

Blood pressure _____

Urine (sugar, protein?) _____

Any effacement or dilation? _____

Other tests? _____

About That Disappearing Waist

Maybe it's time to stop measuring my so-called waist and th

thigh-hopeful-of-remaining-unchanged . . . . and just have

baby! (Or, if I'm truly brave, I can jot the waist, _____

inches, and thigh, _____ inches, here.)

Comments or Instructions from My Care Giver(s):

"Were you planning on having a baby at some point?"

_____

_____

_____

Questions I Want to Remember to Ask:

"Didn't you tell me that the baby comes out eventually??"

_____

_____

_____

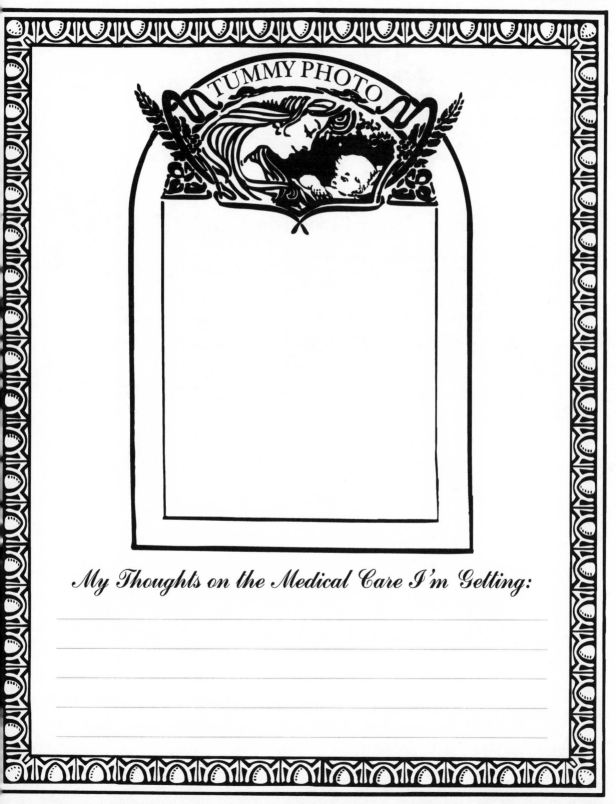

TUMMY PHOTO

My Thoughts on the Medical Care I'm Getting:

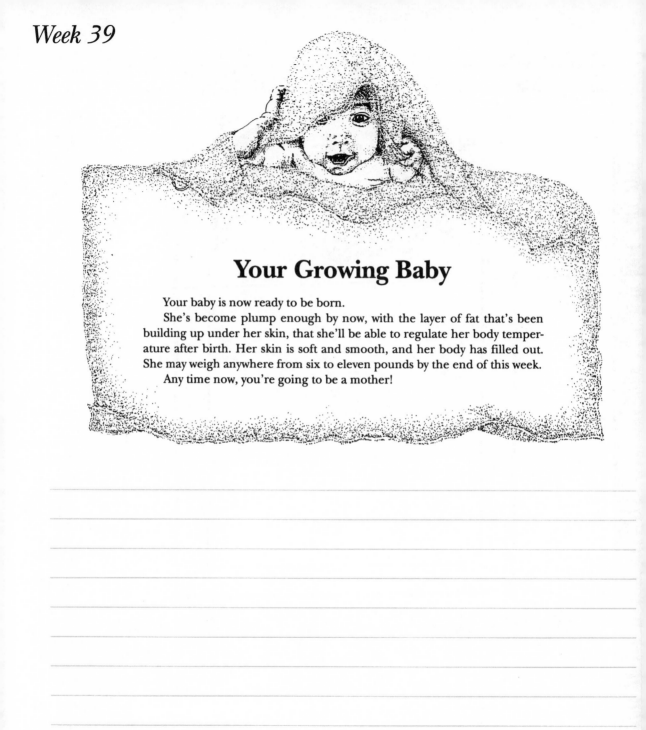

Your Growing Baby

Your baby is now ready to be born.

She's become plump enough by now, with the layer of fat that's been building up under her skin, that she'll be able to regulate her body temperature after birth. Her skin is soft and smooth, and her body has filled out. She may weigh anywhere from six to eleven pounds by the end of this week.

Any time now, you're going to be a mother!

My Thoughts

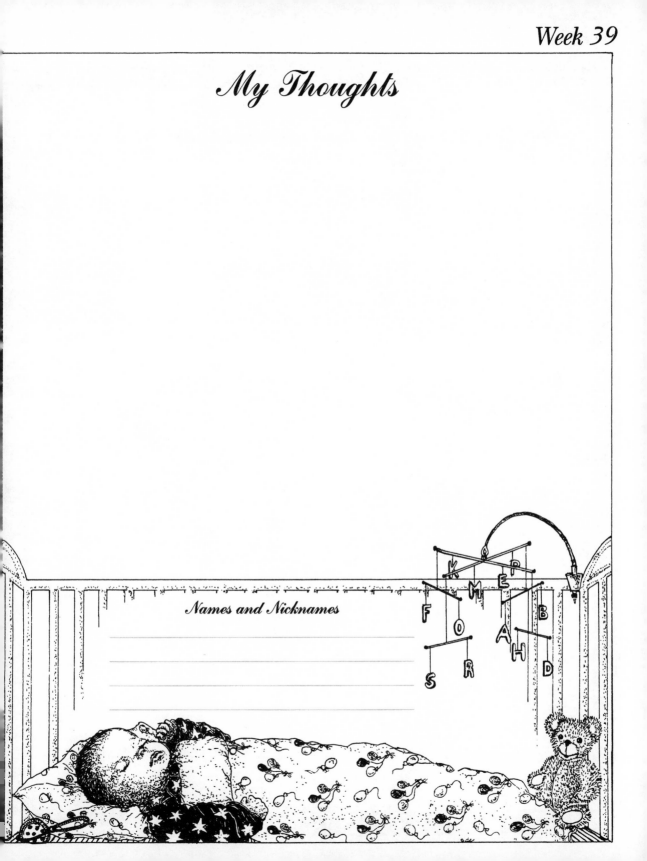

Names and Nicknames

What has pregnancy taught me about patience?

My Dreams

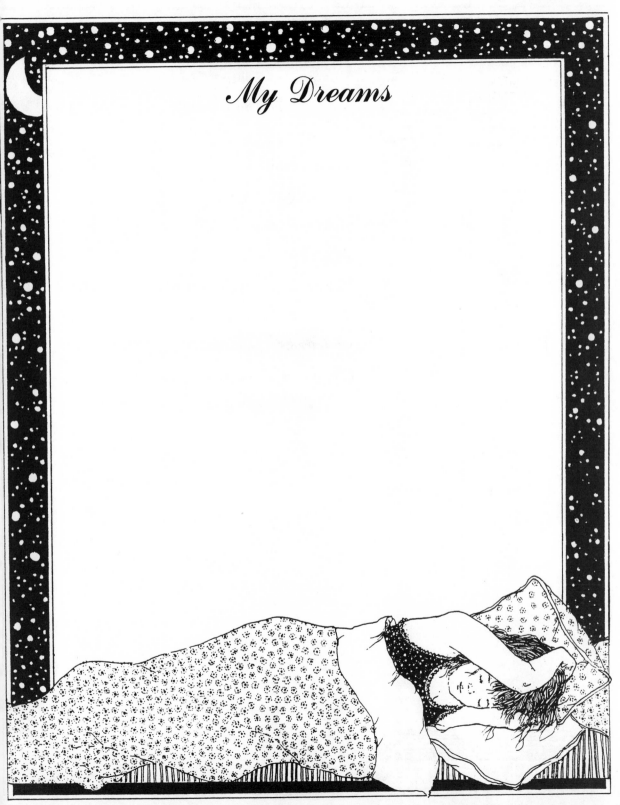

My (39 Week) Doctor Visit

Weight _____ lbs.

Pounds gained since last visit _____ lbs.

Fundal height _____

Blood pressure _____

Urine (sugar, protein?) _____

Effacement or dilation? _____

Other tests? _____

Measurements of Parts of What Used to Be My Body

If I still have the courage or energy to measure any part of me,

this is the space for it! Waist _____ Thigh _____ .

Comments or Instructions from My Care Giver(s):

_____

_____

_____

_____

Questions I Want to Remember to Ask:

"Am I going to be permanently pregnant?"

_____

_____

_____

_____

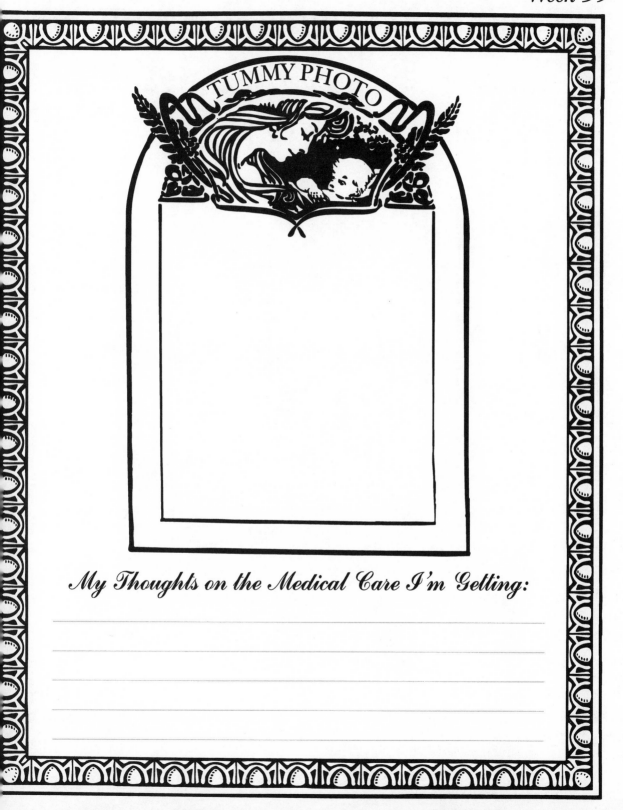

TUMMY PHOTO

My Thoughts on the Medical Care I'm Getting:

_____
_____
_____
_____
_____

How soon after the birth will I look for a scale?! What new feelings do I have about my baby?

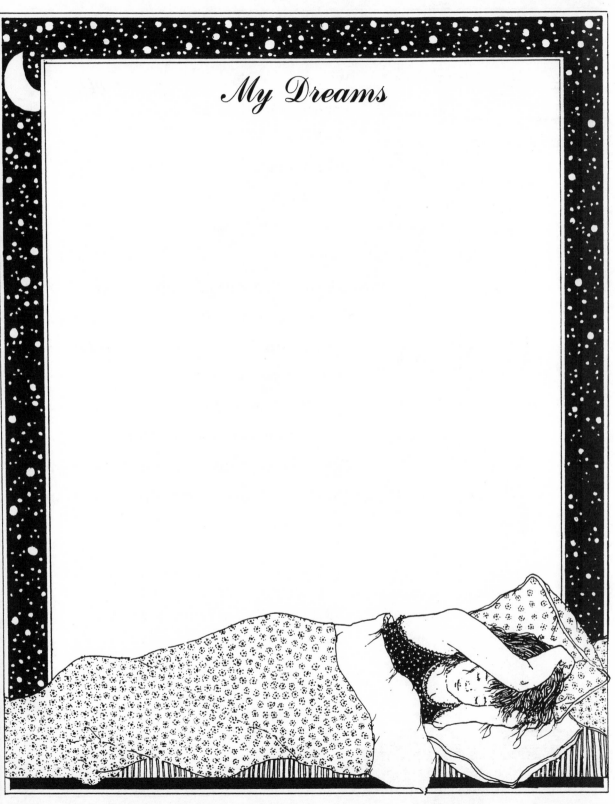

My Dreams

My (40 Week) Doctor Visit

Weight _____ lbs.

Pounds gained since last visit _____ lbs.

Fundal height _____

Blood pressure _____

Urine (sugar, protein?) _____

Effacement or dilation? _____

Other tests? _____

Who Are We Kidding about Measurements?!

I've given up on this stuff about waist measurement! I can't even reach that far around my middle or bend over enough to reach my thigh! I just want to have a baby, for heaven's sake!! (But maybe just for posterity, my middle now measures _____ inches around, and my thigh is _____.)

Comments or Instructions from My Care Giver(s):

"No offense, but we're kind of sick of seeing you in here."

....

....

Questions I Want to Remember to Ask:

"Ditto."

....

....

....

....

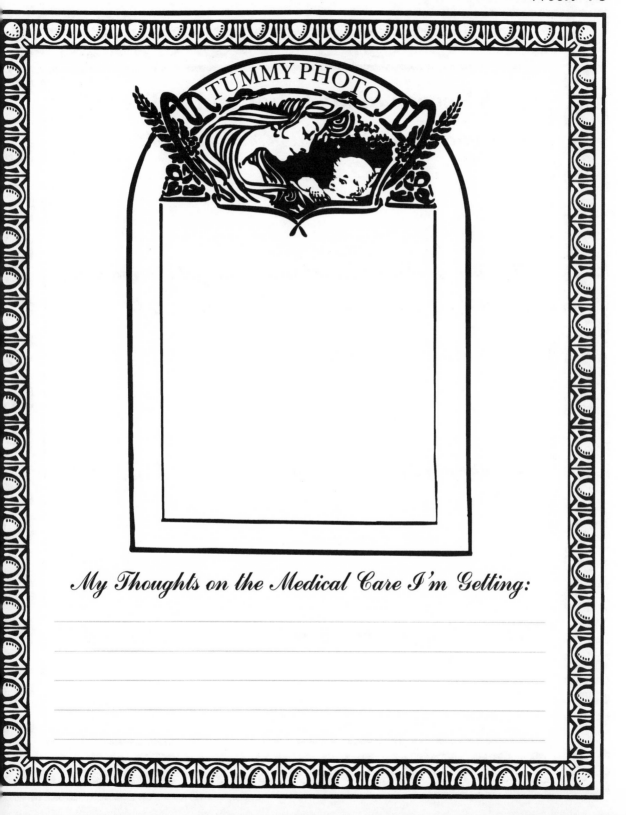

TUMMY PHOTO

My Thoughts on the Medical Care I'm Getting:

A Record of My Labor and Delivery

When and where did my contractions start?

What was my reaction when I realized the moment of truth had arrived and I was really in labor?

How did my husband react when I told him?

Did I call anyone else to let them know "this was it"?

How many minutes apart were the contractions when I called the doctor or hospital?

_____

_____

_____

Did the mucus plug come out? Did my water break? Where was I when it happened?

_____

_____

_____

How long did I stay at home before going to the hospital?

_____

_____

_____

What happened once I got to the hospital?

What was the last thing I ate before labor began?

Did I find the childbirth training helpful? What was the most/least effective technique I learned?

Was I satisfied with my doctor? When did he or she get to the hospital, and how long did the doctor stay?

How many hours of labor were there before I reached transition and was told it wouldn't be much longer?

_____
_____
_____
_____

And how much longer after transition until I was fully dilated or had the urge to push?

_____
_____
_____
_____

If I had a cesarean, what information or feelings do I want to include here? _____

_____
_____
_____
_____

How long did I push? _____
_____
_____
_____
_____

Did I see the baby's head crowning—and how did it
make me feel? _____
_____
_____
_____
_____
_____
_____

What were my first thoughts and feelings when I
saw the baby's body coming out of me?
_____
_____
_____
_____
_____
_____

Who cut the umbilical cord?

What feelings did I have when she was put into my arms?

How did I feel the first time I saw my husband holding our baby?

How were the nurses and other hospital staff? Was anyone especially supportive and helpful?

_____

_____

_____

_____

What would I like to say to my child about his birth, when he is old enough to understand?

_____

_____

_____

_____

_____

Did I have any thoughts about my mother during the labor and delivery? _____

_____

_____

_____

_____

What was the biggest surprise of giving birth?

_____

_____

_____

What part of the experience was very different from what I'd anticipated? _____

_____

_____

_____

Is there anything I wish I'd been better prepared for?

_____

_____

_____

What advice about childbirth would I give to someone else? _____

_____

_____

Baby's Day of Birth Memories

What was the headline in the newspaper? (You can paste it on the "Mementos Page" facing this.)

Who first held the baby? Who was she passed to next?

Who cut the umbilical cord?

Did she cry when she came out? (How loudly and for how long?!)

What was the first thing said about the baby when she was born, and who said it?

Did anyone take photos or videotape the birth? (You can paste a newborn photo on the "Mementos Page" facing this.)

To whom did you make the first phone call?

Which Relative Did the Baby Resemble and Why?

Who did the baby resemble at birth?

Whose nose?

Whose eyes?

Whose chin?

Whose hair? (Did she *have* any hair??)

Mementos of Our Baby's Day of Birth

Life After Birth—The First Month

In what ways is my new life different from what I imagined it would be?

_____

_____

_____

_____

_____

_____

_____

_____

_____

_____

_____

_____

_____

_____

_____

_____

How is my baby different than I expected?

_____

_____

_____

_____

_____

_____

_____

_____

What feelings do I have about the way I've decided to feed my baby?

_____

_____

_____

_____

_____

_____

The Second Month of My New Life

What information about pregnancy or childbirth do I wish other mothers had given me?

What advice would I give about childbirth and new motherhood to someone close to me?

My Third Month of "Life with Baby"

What are the best parts of new motherhood?

_____

_____

What are my favorite times of the day?

_____

_____

What about my baby give me the most pleasure?

_____

_____

What do I love most about my partner as a father?

_____

_____

_____

_____

_____

What are the worst parts of being a mother?

_____

_____

What's been the hardest adjustment for me?

_____

_____

_____

What do I resent?

_____

_____

What worries or guilt do I have?

_____

_____

_____

What do I miss most about my life-before-baby?

_____

_____

_____

Your Baby's Astrological Sign

Whether or not you believe in the influence of the planets on peoples' personalities, it can be interesting and fun to know something about the sun sign under which your child is born. Some people believe this information can help you relate better to your child, allowing you to enjoy and understand each other more easily. If you are someone who is a follower of astrology and consults her horoscope, you believe your baby will show characteristics of his sun sign from an early age, which allows you to better understand the baby's personality and tendencies. On the other hand, you may think astrology is hogwash! Do what you want with the following information about your child's sign of the zodiac— look at it seriously, with amusement, with skepticism, or just with curiosity!

Each sign of the zodiac has an element associated with it (earth, air, fire, or water) that helps to define its nature. The air signs (Libra, Gemini, and Aquarius) are basically signs of the mind or intellect. The water signs (Cancer, Pisces, and Scorpio) are the emotional ones. Earth signs (Taurus, Virgo, and Capricorn) are practical and down-to-earth. Fire signs (Aries, Sagittarius, and Leo) are aggressive and creative. Books, magazines, and newspapers often use slightly different dates to separate the signs of the zodiac. The dates of sun signs in this diary are the ones most commonly used.

Aquarius
(January 21 to February 18)

The zodiacal gem is the garnet

If you would cherish friendship true,

In Aquarius well you'll do

To wear this gem of warmest hue—

The garnet.

Aquarius is the sign of a baby with insatiable curiosity about everything around him, highly inventive although not necessarily practical. He can also be a dreamer whose impractical idealism or sentimentalism gets in the way of making sound decisions. Aquarians are often considered the most unconventional or unpredictable of all the signs, so the parents of a little Aquarian shouldn't expect things to run smoothly! He can have an obstinate side to his personality, which can become a problem. Aquarians are very intuitive; it may seem your child is able to read your mind. Because Aquarians are perceptive and unusually sensitive to other people's feelings, try to be straightforward and honest with your child, since he'll probably be aware of your feelings or problems anyway. Sometimes Aquarians have trouble showing their own feelings; they may feel affectionate but not feel comfortable expressing it.

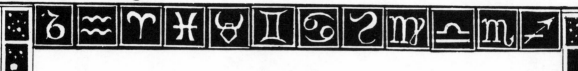

Pisces
(February 19 to March 20)

The zodiacal gem is the amethyst

From passion and from care be kept free

Shall Pisces' children ever be

Who wear so all the world may see

The amethyst.

Pisces is considered an emotional, sensitive, intuitive, and impressionable sign. Pisceans are dreamers who live in a fairy-tale world of their own. There will almost surely be a deep connection and empathy between you and your baby, because her intuitiveness will allow her to understand your moods. Pisceans are affectionate and demonstrative and need to give and receive love. At the same time, they're often basically shy, so let your child dictate how comfortable she is with strangers or in new social situations. Pisceans are also born actors and mimics, so that desire to perform may override her shyness.

Aries
(March 21 to April 20)

The zodiacal gem is the bloodstone

Who on this world of ours his eyes

In Aries opens shall be wise

If always on his hand there lies

A bloodstone.

Ariens are energetic, assertive, and self-expressive, so don't worry about whether your baby can communicate his feelings to you! On the contrary, you may worry if you'll ever again have a chance to express *your* needs! You can be pretty sure that from the moment your little Aries enters your home, he will make it his own. Ariens are enthusiastic and dauntless, without any patience for other people's more cautious approaches. His natural optimism and recklessness with time, energy, and material things often means that an Aries makes the impossible come true. The ruling planet of Aries is Mars, the god of war in mythology, and this influence may give your child a tendency to put up his dukes, although if he does get angry, it's over in a flash. The best way to deal with his combative edge is not to engage it; try not to arbitrarily force your child to do something. Explanation or negotiation will get you further with an Arien than battling things out head to head.

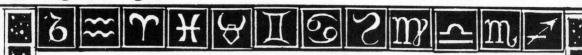

Taurus
(April 21 to May 21)

The zodiacal gem is the sapphire

If on your hand this stone you bind,

You in Taurus born will find

'Twill cure diseases of the mind,

The sapphire.

A Taurean child will be a solid citizen: patient, practical, steadfast, and restrained. A Taurus can be passive in accepting what life hands out, but at the same time have a determined mind. A little Taurean will probably be an easy baby, although the stubborn side of her nature may emerge if you want to do something when she's not in the mood. A Taurus child can be well behaved and a pleasure to raise as long as you understand her. You can avoid battles of will and tantrums with your child if your demands are rational; a Taurean child is less likely to be resistant if you give explanations for your requests. More than most children, Taureans want to know "why" before they go along with the wishes of others. Taureans are affectionate babies who love to be hugged and kissed. A happy home is an asset for any baby but is especially important to a Taurus, who is more sensitive than her calm exterior may indicate. A home that is peaceful and harmonious will bring out the best in your child since it is the foundation for her sense of security and her easygoing, sweet nature.

Gemini
(May 22 to June 22)

The zodiacal gem is the agate

Gemini's children health and wealth command,

And all the ills of age withstand,

Who wear their rings on either hand

Of agate.

Gemini, the sign of the twins, means that you should expect the unexpected—inconsistency is a trademark of this sign. A Gemini baby has a colorful imagination, enormous energy, and a curiosity about the world around him that should keep you on your toes. His desire for a variety of experiences means he adapts easily to new people and places, but with his inquiring mind, a Gemini finds it boring to have a set routine. Your child will need plenty of stimulation, yet Geminis aren't usually good at focusing or concentrating, so you can help your child by directing his imagination and intellectual abilities.

Cancer
(June 23 to July 23)

The zodiacal gem is the emerald

If born in Cancer's sign, they say,

Your life will joyful be always,

If you take with you on your way

An emerald.

Sensitivity, imagination, and a compassion for others are the hallmarks of a Cancer. Your baby craves love and cuddling and will also show a great deal of love toward you. Your child's loving appreciation of everything you do will probably override any difficulties you have adapting to her emotionality. Cancers are vulnerable and sensitive, with feelings that can easily be hurt if they feel misunderstood or unloved. Your child will also probably be shy, so will need your reassurance when it's time to leave the security of home and meet new people in new places. She can seem to be easygoing, but she won't react well to unexpected changes. It's natural for a Cancer to be moody, for a smile to turn to tears, so don't overreact to her tearful or irritable moments.

Leo
(July 24 to August 23)

The zodiacal gem is the onyx

When youth to manhood shall have grown,

Under Leo born and lone

'Twill have lived but for this tone,

The onyx.

Leo's symbol is a lion . . . so you shouldn't be surprised that your child is self-assertive! You'd better be ready to keep up, because your little Leo will have high spirits and inexhaustible energy. The ruling planet of Leo is the sun, which reflects in a Leo's personality: sunny and optimistic, with a big heart. Yet dignity and pride are fundamental to a Leo, who won't be content until she gets the approval and attention she needs. Life will be easier if you teach your little Leo that she is not the sun around whom everyone else revolves! Underneath the powerful Leo is a sweet, vulnerable person who can feel crushed if she feels disapproval, and your little Leo will be an easy child once she realizes who's in charge.

Virgo
(August 24 to September 23)

The zodiacal gem is the carnelian

Success will bless whate'er you do,

Through Virgo's sign, if only you

Place on your hand her own gem true,

Carnelian.

Virgo is the critic of the zodiac (so don't be surprised if your Virgo baby lets you know the right way to put on the diaper!). Virgoans are bright and imaginative, with an intellectual quickness and the verbal skills to win any argument. He may have a hard time showing his love or appreciation and may express his feelings in a more subtle way. A Virgoan enjoys hard work and dedicates himself to a task; he is often successful, because he is tenacious where others give up. At the same time a Virgo can be insecure and may need reassurance that he isn't second best, especially if you have other children. Be aware of your Virgo's vulnerabilities, such as his shyness around strangers, his times of feeling insecure, or his tendency to worry about all the things that might go wrong.

Libra
(September 24 to October 23)

The zodiacal gem is the chrysolite

Through Libra's sign it is quite well

To free yourself from evil spell,

For in her gem surcease doth dwell,

The chrysolite.

A Libran is one of the most good-natured signs in the zodiac. Your child will be adaptable, eager to be kind and to have harmony around her. A sense of order based on fairness and truth is essential to the Libra personality. Librans are ruled by Venus, goddess of love, and she may seem to be born with an irresistible smile on her little face that can melt hearts! A quirk of Librans is that they cannot make decisions easily. Too many choices are difficult for her, and from an early age you may have to guide your child in making up her mind. You'll need to be patient with your Libran's indecisiveness, which is a small price to pay for her lovely disposition.

Scorpio
(October 24 to November 23)

The zodiacal gem is the beryl

Through Scorpio this gem so fair

Is that which everyone should wear,

Or tears of sad repentance bear—

The beryl.

A Scorpio is a complex person, with strength of character that will be evident even when your baby is still very small. Scorpios are emotionally intense, with a definite personality. A Scorpio child can be temperamental and poised for a tantrum if he doesn't get his own way, so it's up to you to set limits. Developing an understanding and respect for what makes your little fellow tick should make for family compatibility. Scorpios can be highly intuitive: your child will probably know if something is bothering you just from your tone of voice or the look in your eyes. Yet a Scorpio needs privacy and tends to be secretive, so it probably won't be so easy for you to know your child's innermost thoughts (unless, of course, you're a Scorpio, too!).

Sagittarius
(November 24 to December 22)

The zodiacal sign is the topaz

Who first comes to this world below

Under Sagittarius should know

That their true gem should ever show

The topaz.

    Mentally and physically, this sign is the explorer of the zodiac, so you won't have much rest as soon as your baby can move around! Sagittarians adapt easily to new situations, so traveling or moving with a Sagittarius child will be a pleasure. Sagittarians are energetic and good at expressing and asserting themselves. Along with her inborn independence and self-assurance, she will also be a devoted friend who is popular with others. Your Sagittarian will be friendly and relaxed, which will make it easy to overlook her less pleasant characteristic, which is a tendency to be argumentative.

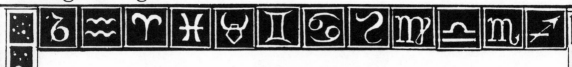

Capricorn
(December 23 to January 20)

The zodiacal gem is the ruby

Those who live in Capricorn

No trouble shall their brows adorn

If they this glowing gem have worn,

The ruby.

    Capricorns are often thought of as old souls, so you may have a baby with a wise head on little shoulders. He may seem so grown-up and responsible that it's a pleasure for you, so remember to encourage him to lighten up and enjoy being a child! He may seem to take life too seriously, and laughing off mistakes or obstacles is not something he can do without your help. Those born under this sign are cautious by nature, and they keep their cards close to the vest. A Capricorn likes a structure to his life, and he might be most comfortable if you follow a set routine in how you handle, bathe, and feed him. Emotional security is especially important to Capricorns, and a sense of harmony and order in the family. If there are family problems, your Capricorn child may not exhibit his sensitivity outwardly, but he will pick up on the tensions and be disturbed by them.